PEOPLE MEDICINE

PEOPLE MEDICINE

A Frugal Physician
prescribes
Common Sense and Enthusiasm

by
Robert McNary MD

PEOPLE MEDICINE
A Frugal Physician Prescribes Common Sense and Enthusiasm

Copyright 2011 by Robert McNary All Rights Reserved

Manufactured in the United States of America

Editorial Assistance by
Charlotte McDevitt
Tracy Deliman
Nicolas Ortiz Cue

Cover and layout by
Curt Perkins / Electric Avenue Nashville

Published by
The Portable School Press
theportableschool@gmail.com
www.peoplemedicine.net

PEOPLE MEDICINE
A Frugal Physician prescribes Common Sense and Enthusiasm

Part 1 - Common Sense

Foreword
Common Sense and Enthusiasm
Dead or Alive?
Practicing Medicine
Insuring Care?
Bizness
Working in Pain
Fear Not
Hoofbeats
Scientific Medicine
Routine Tests
Normal?
Xray! Xray! Read All About It
Rocket Science
Clinic Visits
Hospital Time
Pen Light
Germs and Disease
The Life That Lives on Man
Bigger Bugs & Bigger People
Playing Catch
What Do We Really Know?
In the Name of . . .
Name Your Poison
Disease Rights
Purple Pills & Magic Bullets
Cut to Cure
Fighting Disease, Saving Lives

Part 2 - Enthusiasm

Medical Heresy
Good Medicine, Bad Medicine
Diagnosis, Disease and Dis-ease
Anything Can Cause Anything
Anything Can Cure Anything
Teaching and Learning
Lip Service
Buddha Ears
Good Hand
Touching Experiences
Holy Presence
House Calls
Family Practice
Home Remedies
The Whole Works
The Body Electric
The Mind Body
True Psychology
Depth Physiology
Cause and Effect
Healing Times
The Gift of Disease
Patients of Job
Going the Distance
Temples of Healing
Bleeding Always Stops
An Inside Job
The Greatest Healer

Afterword and Appendices

Dedicated to the Spirit of HPB

~ ~ ~ ~ ~

*"The progressive thinking of one era
is the common sense of the next."*
Matthew Arnold

*"Every great and commanding movement in the annals
of the world is the triumph of enthusiasm."*
Ralph Waldo Emerson

"First, do no harm."
Hippocrates

Foreword

The idea for this book arose after a brief encounter at the grocery store. I ran into Dwight Thompson. Dwight is our local Physician Assistant, a kind-hearted man with many years in rural practice. He is also a thinker.

Once in a while we run into each other and compare notes for a few moments. That day, we focused on the small town hospital's recent loss of its only full-time, long-term physicians - a husband and wife team. As they were heading back to their home state of Michigan, the citizenry and hospital staff were wondering and worrying about the future of the hospital, clinic and nursing home.

Dwight said something like, "Things sure have changed in our time. It's harder and harder to keep a small town hospital running. Costs are so high for our facility and for our patients."

The conversation turned to what health care providers do and do not know about costs of tests and treatments they recommend. Dwight admitted he wasn't well informed on the former. We both related that we had NEVER had classes in our training on medical care costs. It just wasn't considered necessary.

However, technology is coming to the rescue - to a degree. Dwight pulled out his Blackberry and ran a program which showed the costs of common prescription drugs. He quickly pointed out one which was priced at ten dollars a pill. That was hardly top price. My teeth dropped, not having purchased any kind of medication in decades. "How does anyone afford it?"

Obviously, many people can't afford modern medicine which has prompted politicians and legislators to try to "fix" the medical care system. But, the first question also begets others like:

Will reformed medicine be more affordable than what we have?
Will the new version just be more of the present system?
Is our current system as good as generally thought?
Are the costs of medical intervention equal to the benefits?
What about the side effects, accidents, negligence, malpractice?

What about alternatives, prevention, traditional practices?
Is it possible to go beyond the current medical paradigm?

This book evolved from the angle of frugality, conservation and common sense. But, it has gathered a life of its own and has grown to address the whole of the modern medical system.

Though a small volume, PEOPLE MEDICINE considers not just saving medical money but also the dogmas of medical training, the reliance on tests and technology, the religion of science, the "bigger is better" concept, competence vs. care, and more. The book does not just poke and prod on problems and shortcomings, but suggests real life possibilities for change and improvement.

If you read between the lines, A Frugal Physician can help YOU conserve resources, ask the right questions, gain perspective, learn about health and disease, and better understand the system in which you place your body and your hopes. It can also teach you how to recognize the caring, conscious people you need when you are ill or injured.

Note I: This book is meant to bring information, ideas, and maybe a little inspiration to the table regarding modern medicine and healing. To accomplish that aim, it is necessary to look at the defects, errors, and problems in the present system. COMMON SENSE helps out here.

This process leads us to consider BETTER WAYS, things about which we can show ENTHUSIASM. But at the same time, the author wants the reader to remember that over all, physicians and nurses have been and are hard working, caring and unstinting in their efforts to aid and comfort their fellow beings. Their sincerity and desire to be of service are credits to the human race. They have taken on the challenges of disease and pain, trauma and injury and made sacrifices for the betterment of their brothers and sisters. They deserve honor and thanks for bringing us this far.

Yet, medicine and its practitioners have not kept pace with the illnesses and problems of the times as well as the world of deep and growing knowledge which surrounds us. We continue to fight old diseases with stale ideas and limited perspectives. It is time to make substantial changes in medical practice which fit with the people and the era.

Note II: One reviewer has called a number of the thoughts and themes in the book extreme. There is truth to the suggestion. Let the reader beware, but also consider the real possibility that modern medicine may be itself the greater extreme.

Note III: Most medical professors and mentors retain their real names in the book. Innocent friends as well as the potentially "guilty" who may take offense have been given pseudonyms.

Note IV: "All medicine is anecdotal." Since every person is unique, every illness and injury is as well. Statistics do not mean much in individual situations. But stories may pass on real value to those who are open to them. Statistics are not known for their healing ability, but a well told tale may revive or rejuvenate, invigorate or inspire.

Note V: Here are some thoughts on the word Frugal. It may be a more inclusive word than the reader has imagined. Like many words, Frugal (derived from the Latin *frugalis* for virtuous, after *frux* for fruit) has lots of meanings. We can use the word as a standard and guidepost, considering it in its best light to mean:

careful	provident
caring	prudent
conserving	sage
disciplined	sensible
economical	saving
efficient	sparing
mature	thrifty
parsimonious	unwasteful
practical	wary
preserving	wise

PART I: COMMON SENSE

Common Sense and Enthusiasm

Shortly after completing the first clinical rotation of my junior year in medical school, I received an "invitation" to meet with Senior Physician Dr. Walter Kirkendall, the Chief of Internal Medicine for the Hermann Hospital and the whole medical school (University of Texas Medical School at Houston). I had no idea what prompted the summons, but quickly found out once I stopped into his office.

Kirkendall was an aging internist, a big guy in a long white coat with professorial glasses sliding down over his nose. He was a looming authority figure and I was just a tyro. Still, he was neither welcoming nor unkind. Just matter of fact. He didn't ask me to sit down. He simply got to the point. "Your evaluation for your first rotation on Medicine was not very good. It concludes, 'Student lacks common sense and enthusiasm.' Let's see that you do better in this next round. I don't want to hear anything about a repeat performance."

Short and sweet. Well, not really sweet. Not harsh either. Dr. Kirkendall added something to the effect that the next evaluation would have to show improvement - or else.

The first two years of medical school were (and still are) largely classroom work, sitting for hours listening to generally boring, uninspired lectures and speakers. (If I had to do it over again, I would skip practically all classes, read the texts which I would anyway, and find real life experiences to fill the time I "should" be in the classroom.)

A common refrain in the Texas Medical Center and other points of medical training was "Them that can do, do. Them that can't do, teach." I couldn't object much. Actually, I came to the conclusion that the quality of teaching I sat through for almost two decades of my life had gotten worse instead of better as my education progressed to "higher" levels.

An anecdote about a notorious professor at our neighboring school,

Baylor College of Medicine, circulated freely if not accurately. Most certainly it carried savory grains of truth. Apparently, the medical man directed a course to a large group (200+) in an amphitheater-style auditorium. (I was in one of the first classes of UTMSH and our group of 52 had the "luck" to be taught for two years in cramped makeshift classrooms on the 11th and 12th floor of Center Pavilion Hospital, then on the edge of Texas Medical Center.) While his lectures were poorly received, the instructor didn't pay heed. His talks droned on and on. But, what was a student to do?

Medical people - even students - are rarely spontaneous or innovative, but one student took it upon himself to make a statement for the whole class. His friends helped him move a couch into the auditorium prior to a lecture session. They placed it strategically at the base of the amphitheater directly in front of the long counter behind which lecturers were wont to speak and scribble on the equally long blackboards covering the rear wall.

That day as the professor's drone became oppressive, the brave young student quietly left his seat and stretched out on the couch. He was soon asleep. The professor either didn't notice or didn't care. Surely, the students must have found it difficult to keep from bursting out in laughter.

I can count on one hand the number of interesting professors and classes we had in those first two years - and still have fingers left over. Only one instructor comes to mind at the present moment. That is Dr. Guillermo Nottebohm. The Argentine firecracker was a nephrologist (kidney specialist) who taught classes on internal medicine. He was dynamic, devoted to his work and specialty. He moved around, tried to engage the people in the seats, and told pertinent or at least provocative stories. While he didn't have "new" information for us, he presented his classes with some energy and excitement.

I recall his recurring pronouncement given out when students said they hadn't gotten their reading or assignment done. Spoken with his spicy Spanish accent, he said, "My young man, you really have no excuse. There is no requirement for medical students to get sleep. So, you certainly had time to get this work done."

Dr. Nottebohm and a bare few others helped us survive those grueling hours in our tiny, stuffy classroom. Fortunately even in the first med school years, we did get away for a few hours each week for one kind of practicum or another. When we reached the third year, everyone was quite relieved. Our butt-numbing classroom hours were slashed to a minimum.

We then spent practically all our time on one ward/service or another - six weeks at a stint. The ward team usually consisted of an attending physician who was the titular head of the group and appeared at his/her own discretion. Some did daily, others on occasion. Generally, s/he handed responsibilities over to a resident physician and an intern. Medical students pulled up the rear and took directions and orders from everyone. We did physical exams and procedures, chased test results, made regular rounds checking on patients, attended our mentors' needs and whims, acted as go-betweens, and did whatever other gopher work was delegated to us.

My first rotation was on the Cancer Ward at the Hermann (University) Hospital. It was a sad and depressing place for patients and workers alike. The prognosis for most patients was less than hopeful. When my "cancer rounds" were over, I thought I had done the work and followed the program. But, I learned otherwise from Dr. Kirkendall. I had opened my mouth one too many times.

Dr. John Rogers, the Medical Resident on the Cancer Ward, was tightly wound and equally bound to the medical orthodoxy. He had obviously not liked my pointed questions, especially when I showed I was unconvinced as to the value of some of the treatments - antibiotics and steroids, steroids and antibiotics - which we doled out so frequently and freely.

On one occasion, I remember Rogers calling me a "therapeutic nihilist." Suggesting that I wasn't enthusiastic about any medical methods. He wasn't far from the truth.

By that time, I had developed a questioning eye and skeptical opinion about many things. I also had studied enough on my own about other schools of medicine, traditions and alternatives to object, at least inwardly, to many teachings we were expected to accept at face value. Supplemented by my several years of experience as medical corpsman, Xray assistant, vocational nurse, and medical technologist, I had a broad knowledge base larger than most medical students and as wide as many resident physicians.

I found that the modern medical guild, probably like older ones, does not appreciate alternative thinking. When I was in Uncle Sam's Army, we were told, "There's the right way, the wrong way, and the Army way." There's a Medical way, as well.

Chief Resident Rogers also took it quite personally when patients died, on one occasion painfully and blatantly blaming the nurses. Death in the medical system is too often seen as a failure. And with failure, someone needs to take the blame.

But, really! People die, like cancer patients on cancer wards.

Nonetheless, MY basic problem was "lack of common sense and enthusiasm." I admit that I most surely must have frowned inwardly as well as questioned more than was "right for a newby." I didn't have the common sense to keep my mouth shut when I couldn't be clearly enthusiastic about standard methods.

I tried to button my lip more the second time around than the first. (Not an easy task.) But, that second rotation went much better - or, again, so I thought - at St. Joseph's Hospital which was located in downtown Houston away from the Texas Medical Center. Dr. Jim Peterson, the head resident, was decidedly laid back. He wasn't out to shine, just get the job done, take care of people, and move along the medical corridor. The number two man was an OB-GYN intern who tried to lighten the load with laughter. Further, we were working on a general medical ward. Death was not the constant daily threat as it had been at the Hermann cancer ward.

I did my work, followed the protocols, and made no waves regarding patient care. So, I was not entirely surprised that there was no further word from Dr. Kirkendall. However, some weeks after finishing that rotation, my medical student partner at St. Joseph's let me know, "The word is that they lost the evaluations Peterson wrote for us!" Maybe that was for the good. I will never know.

I do know that, then and more so now, common sense and

enthusiasm are essential to a well-rounded life as well as for health and healing. Despite the seeming opposition of the terms, the two might fit nicely on a crest designed for a Frugal Physician.

I have to stop here because I can't help but think that we humans are prone to project our shortcomings on others. I was accused of lacking common sense and enthusiasm. I have since admitted the truth of the accusation. I wonder if medicine and its practitioners can stand up to that accusation as well. My experiences of Kirkendall and Rogers suggested them to be neither particularly common sensical nor enthusiastic.

Much of modern living seems to avoid common sense: "Just follow the regular program." Express your enthusiasm for something extraordinary: "Hold your horses." Object to the status quo: "You are upsetting peace and decorum."

The same ethos seems to hold sway in the corridors of medical institutions most everywhere. Yet, medicine and modernity must find room again for common sense and enthusiasm. I suggest that they are two of the keys which will open the gates to further layers of growth and understanding in the coming era.

COMMON SENSE is a stabilizing force necessary for all of us, whatever our pursuits and interests. "Common problems call for common sense." Common sense suggests mental balance, the gift of discrimination, and rational perspective. It points to the HEAD - a clear one.

Simple approaches and measures should suffice to deal with most medical problems. They have in times past, in less developed parts of the world, and even now with many who don't readily go along with the medical orthodoxy.

Medicine seems to respond: "Things are not so simple as you might think. We have developed protocols and practices which have proven generally effective over the years. We apply our highly technical and tested knowledge toward the betterment of our patients and society."

Medicine and physicians wish us to believe their works to be arcane and understandable to only the trained and certified. Medicine has long been mystified so as to empower physicians and make patients and public dependent. The whole of life has been medicalized in the words of Ivan Illich (*Medical Nemesis*). Wise Physicians know and act otherwise to share knowledge, promote health and level the field.

ENTHUSIASM, coming from the Greek *en theos* and meaning in God, inspired by God - points to energies of the HEART. To the author, enthusiasm hints at being on fire, devoted to an unselfish, universal cause. Enthusiasm opens us to the deeper parts of our humanity, world, and life.

Medicine replies: "Our work is to tend and repair the human body. We know nothing of the soul or God. That is outside of our element. If a patient needs God, call the chaplain."

Despite such objections, the forces of common sense and enthusiasm can help expand the dimensions of modern medical care beyond its present limited confines. One bringing down-to-earth focus and the other reaching for everpresent hidden possibilities. "Feet on the ground and head in the heavens."

We are all so built - more or less. Why can't the future medicine grow in that direction? One Frugal Physician believes so. "Once a physician, always a physician."

Maybe Drs. Rogers and Kirkendall did me (us) a real favor by helping to point out these fundamental forces which can be used to direct our steps in the ways of A Frugal Physician.

In the following pages, we will draw on common sense to look at the present state of medicine. Enthusiasm will arise later as we consider brighter and better ways which can lead all of us from medicine to healing.

The epithet "frugal physician" is an oxymoron just as in a similar vein, common sense and enthusiasm make for a combination of near opposites. However, both can make for useful pairs.

Here are a few other medical oxymorons, most of which we will consider as we go along:

health insurance
preventive medicine
health care
fixing health care

cutting to cure
therapeutic tests
medical practice
scientific medicine

Putting Frugal and Physician together is clearly unusual and uncommon. A quick search at Google gives a paltry string of 200 citations out of billions of web pages. "Frugal physician" references mostly point to ways for physicians to save money and resources in their offices or how to adjust their lifestyles at home. A large share of results are given for Frugal Physician Medical Supplies, a name brand. There is nary a word about medical people helping their patients to save money.

In the modern world, the practice of medicine very often mandates substantial costs. Even to walk into a medical office necessitates leaving several large bills on the counter or writing a good sized check.

"Physicians are not taught to save money. They are taught to save lives." I just made that one up, but it seems a relative medical truism in the common era. (Saving lives is another oxymoron we will survey later.)

Medical people need to know that financial health and physical health go hand in hand. One reflects the other very commonly and is dependent on the other more than is often apparent. That is a basic understanding for a Frugal Physician.

With expensive tests and technology, pills and procedures taking over larger and larger swaths of medicine, parsimony in health care is almost unknown. It was known and common in the past. The time is surely opportune for a return to rational and wise medical care. Such may become infectious and break out in the rest of society.

Common sense and enthusiasm may help us achieve such a desirable destination. Frugal Physicians must help bring that into being. Money will be saved, resources conserved, and waste reduced. At the same time, human beings will be enabled to relate to each other more directly and wholesomely. Health and healing will rise like the phoenix out of the old and decrepit medical model.

Dead or Alive?

Common sense is surely still alive. Certainly, the common folk still have some common sense. Still, it's just not as COMMON as it once was and harder to find in some places. Many forces in modern life make it more and more difficult to live simply, wisely, and economically.

In his 1995 book *The Death of Common Sense*, Philip K. Howard explains how our modern legalistic way of looking at things twists us around and makes common sense much less common. I heard New York City lawyer Howard on the radio a few years ago and was duly impressed with his message. The sixteen years since he wrote his book haven't improved the general state of common sense in the world and more particularly in our part of it.

Subtitling his book *How Law is Suffocating America*, Howard says that laws and lawyers and legislators are making it very hard for people to live normal lives. Businesses and consumers seem to have the law hanging over their heads at most every turn. "You better not do that or you might get sued." "You'll get into trouble with the government if you don't do this."

The threat of litigation or government intervention is so prevalent that it affects almost every area of our lives. It makes things more expensive because of insurance, police, lawyers, etc. and makes us behave like we are paranoid. And our paranoia continues to grow, especially now with all the hysteria related to terrorists and the War on Terrorism.

One of the arresting stories Mr. Howard told over the radio was about a woman who was shopping in a furniture store when she tripped and broke her ankle. Claiming that the store was at fault, the woman went to court and got a judgment against the business for $79,000. On the surface, the judgment doesn't sound too unusual or totally out of line. But, the kicker was that the woman had tripped over her own child who was crawling on the floor of the store. Can you beat that?!

We might be able to beat it, after all. There is a site on the Internet which has been giving out Stella Awards to "honor" such kinds of events. The Awards were named after the woman (Stella Liebeck) who received a $2.9 million settlement from McDonald's after Stella dropped a cup of hot coffee in her own lap. (Visit stellaawards.com.)

Philip Howard suggests that rules have become a religion. Laws are replacing our humanity. Uniformity is king while diversity is becoming illegal. Bureaucrats rule by relying on codes, laws, and regulations. Our government of laws works against us. Lawyers spend much of their time (and clients' money) involved in adversarial legalisms. Lawsuits are rampant. Thought and judgment have been banished so that we fear government authority.

Most all of these points have bearing on the practice of medicine in our time. Let's take a quick look at some of them.

"Rules have become a religion." All kinds of rules circumscribe medical practice: Laws set down by the government through programs such as Medicare, Medicaid and Social Security; guidelines from insurance companies; standards set by the American Medical Association and the American Hospital Association; and so on. Hospital and clinic administrators literally have REAMS of rules to follow.

Medics aim at Quality Care but often end up meeting guidelines and keeping the closet clean for inspection. The medical situation is akin to standards set by the recent No Child Left Behind Law which create lowest common denominator kinds of schools. Such laws, although well intended, do in fact become "religious dogma" which practitioners, clinics and hospitals must follow. Else they be excommunicated.

I am reminded of a report sent out by my medical school following our 20th year reunion. The main theme going through comments of my old classmates was too much paperwork, too many rules, too much government intervention. Several seasoned physicians hinted at wanting to find another profession.

"Laws are replacing our humanity." In the medical setting, paper work and protocols become more important these days than direct care and timely attention to human concerns for the patient and often for workers in the field. Throughout the medical chain of command, paperwork rules.

There is only so much time in the day to meet all demands. So, mandated rules and attendant forms take precedence. Care is too often determined by squiggles on paper rather than effects in patients' lives.

I remember talking not long ago to an ER doc who complained about paper work and the "cut and paste" process which had then become the pattern for completing required examination forms. In my own case when I was an Army flight surgeon, I was mandated to do rectal exams with every annual flight physical. When paperwork was returned because I hadn't performed the test - thinking it intrusive and unnecessary, I lied and checked the WNL (within normal limits) box. The system accepted my lies.

Quality Assurance has become a numbers game. Hospitals distribute surveys for patients to rate their care according to a Numeric Scale. That seems like another oxymoron to me.

"Let's make Quality Care quantitative," some number cruncher decided. Administrators bought it. Workers use it. People accept it. But, something is surely awry in the process.

"Uniformity is king while diversity is becoming illegal." Well, it has been a long time since the medical profession had room for diversity. Pills and surgery or surgery and pills are the options. If all else fails, the psychiatrist can be consulted.

Innovation is relatively unknown because treatment for labeled and diagnosed diseases are prescribed and alternatives are proscribed. "If you want to use non-standard methods, go back to chiropractic school."

"Bureaucrats rule by relying on codes, laws, and regulations." A common complaint is that bureaucrats of one kind or another and insurance examiners are dictating medical care. There is a certain amount of truth to the statement.

How would patients fare if such influences were not active? Would medical practice really be much different? Most physicians themselves are much more like technicians and bureaucrats than they might ever realize or admit. They regularly follow the same old patterns, like we all do to one degree or another.

Such observation brings up the adage that "Insanity is doing the same thing over and over and expecting a different result." Too often these days, we are allowed no choice. So, the pattern just continues.

"Our government of laws works against us." Attorney Howard's point is that modern laws and rules make "one size fit all." That practice worked for a time. But not forever simply because one size does not fit all.

Times and people have changed. Clearly, our systems have not kept pace.

I am reminded of how patients are so commonly corralled into cancer treatment protocols in which they have to follow their program to the letter. Patients are then more manipulated than really cared for. A whole book surely could be written about patient experiences revolving around destructive cancer therapy laid out in lockstep series of X number of treatments over so many days or weeks so that statistical studies can be done. Their disease and the test program overrule the needs of the patients. How sad, but how regularly accepted.

"Lawyers spend much of their time (and clients' money) involved in adversarial legalisms." This is the "letter of the law" mentality over the "spirit of the law."

Is your physician caring for you or instead battling some diagnosis, disease, label or phantom? Is s/he reading you or just studying the textbook?

How much of your physician's time is spent with you as opposed to your paperwork and tests? Is s/he dealing with numbers and letters or your spirit?

"Lawsuits are rampant." Well, we don't have to go far with this one. Malpractice lawsuits are more and more common. Part of this state of affairs is because lawyers are eager to sue. That's how they make money.

The USA has more lawyers than any other country in the whole world. Not surprising, really. We have one lawyer for every 265 of our citizens. Compare that to the United Kingdom which has one for every 1400 people.

Another part of the problem develops when physicians don't take adequate time with their patients, treat them as another case, and forget that they are dealing with human beings. They set themselves up for errors and problems and lawsuits. Fortunate for them it is that thousands of incidents of error and negligence are overlooked because many patients are quick to forgive even though they take the hit.

But, that is surely changing. Litigiousness is a contagious disease growing with the years. And it is surely catching more and more of the population.

I have often reflected that a lawsuit is one of the few ways for someone in the lower/middle class to take a step up. We used to have opportunities to capture land and space and make our way up the economic ladder. Those options are very limited in the modern world. In the present day, lawsuits, lotteries, and sweepstakes have taken their place.

"Thought and judgment have been banished so that we fear government authority." The key part of this statement revolves around "thought and judgment" which suggests a re-statement of some of the earlier points.

In recent times, I have said much the same but with other less kind words. I look around and think, "People have lost guts and imagination." Sad to say, in the western world, we have become nations of sheep.

We are sheep-like not simply because we aren't capable of more, but largely because our laws and systems have become crystallized and diseased. We continue to prop them up, reinforce them, prevent them from disintegrating and being replaced by new and vital ones. We believe in our staid way of life and have trouble imagining any thing better, although it must be so.

Medicine, like law and government and many other institutions, must open to change. Else they are all doomed to fall apart due to obesity and constipation, short-sightedness and simple ineptitude. Common sense has been replaced by double talk, greed and waste.

Bottom line: The medical system is not alone in its discomfort and ills. Laws and paperwork rule. Doctors and nurses, clinics and hospitals really want to look out for your better health interests. But like the whole country, including the legal system and government, medicine is affected by a long standing and contagious paranoia.

"Better do more tests to CYA (Cover Your Ass)," is a common thought in the profession. Consciously or unconsciously held. CYA is not often voiced aloud, but physicians have it ringing in their ears or drumming on their shoulders. Physicians don't want to miss anything - whether it is for your benefit or theirs - even though it might cost an arm and a leg to find. Yours!

Confronting this sad way of thinking and acting gets harder as the years advance. Common sense seems more and more remote.

Fortunately, it only takes a few to begin making change. A Frugal Physician, motivated by common sense and compassion, thinks first of his/her patients, rather than forms or legalisms. S/he works out of love, not out of fear.

Practicing Medicine

In his book, Philip Howard quotes Grant Gilmore of Yale Law Professor, who had the cheek to say, "The idea of law has been ridiculously oversold." I follow his lead and suggest, "The idea of medicine has been ridiculously oversold."

Actually, it is the *practices* rather than the professions which have been oversold. Both professions are needed and praiseworthy when rightly *practiced*. Both professions seem to have - as my mother might have said - gotten too big for their britches. Making unfounded claims, promoting dubious services, leading patients and clients to believe that they can deliver the undeliverable. Often preaching more than they really *practice*.

Many factors including the several listed in the preceding chapter make it difficult for any physician to *practice* the ART, in whatever way s/he understands his/her calling. How does a doctor make art out of dogma and rules and legalisms? How does a physician create art out of science, especially since art, like business, nutrition, health, is scarcely given time or credence in medical training? Is s/he enabled to address patients' real problems?

The author believes there should be a step beyond *practicing* medicine. Electricians, plumbers and other tradespeople go through defined stages of training and advancement, like apprentice and journeyman, to eventually become masters of their trades. That is not the case with physicians and lawyers, which should give patients and clients some clues.

Generations ago, young physicians apprenticed to older ones. That was in a much different world. Theoretically at least, mastering medicine may have been more possible in those times.

I probably never met a physician who has mastered medicine. Dr. Smythe (see Routine Tests) may have gotten close. The rest of us just practice/d it.

As opposed to common belief, physicians are far from erudite, wise, and all-knowing. For one thing, the trade that they ply is so much more complicated than that of an electrician and plumber. The breadth and depth of plumbing and electrical equipment, installation and repairs are relatively knowable.

Physicians work with living beings who are far more than their bodies which however are the intense focus of physician attention and work. (Does your physician treat you or your body?)

Since we still KNOW only a fraction of human potentials and physicians usually UNDERSTAND human problems only superficially, we may actually have NO Master Physicians. The best you will likely get is one who is caring, growing, learning, changing, willing to listen and explore your person, life situation, and challenges as well as his/her own: A Frugal Physician.

The simple, straightforward fact is that physicians are accomplished at one level or another of Educated Guesswork. That's right. When you go to most any *practitioner* (there is that word again), you are paying money for him/her to *practice* on you. No doubt, s/he has studied long and hard, made the grade passing requisite exams, fulfilled professional commitments and been licensed, certified and insured. But, passing tests and ordering tests are only the standard facets of medical *practice*. Patients are the reason for the *practice* of medicine as well as the point where variation, exceptions, and wonderment set in.

As you will be reminded in these pages many times, every patient is very different from the last. Superficially, a patient may appear to have the same condition or problem as the next. But in a larger sense, that is quite likely to be untrue. And, your physician needs to recognize and honor that.

You and I and all people are unique. Thus we, to a greater or lesser degree, present to clinic and hospital with unique problems and thus unique disease.

Most physicians just scratch the surface when dealing with their fellow human beings. Two hundred years ago, the French writer-philosopher Voltaire hit the nail on the head for his time and into the present, when he said, *"Physicians prescribe drugs of which they know little for diseases of which they know less to patients of which they know absolutely nothing."*

In some respects, things have changed dramatically in the medical world from Voltaire's 18th century. Outwardly, anyway. Physicians have vastly more training, knowledge, and equipment. Scrupulously clean and expensive offices and medical centers. Grand arrays of tests and treatments to choose from. The best that money and technology can provide. Your money.

But with a Big Picture view, we can see - if we have the eyes - that things really haven't advanced in many important parts of medical practice. Let's pick Mr. Voltaire's statement apart.

"Physicians prescribe drugs of which they know little . . ."

Medics have dozens, really hundreds and thousands, more drugs to prescribe than in Voltaire's time. But, pharmaceuticals are expensive, over prescribed, and fraught with adverse reactions and safety concerns.

"But, they know a lot about them?" Yes and No, mostly No. How could your physician really know that much about even a tiny percentage of the available repertory? Or for that matter, know one single medication well unless s/he took it personally for an extended period of time? Or worked with many patients who reported to him/her regularly and faithfully about its internal effects? That is pretty rare. Actually, the physician probably wouldn't like hearing all the details if the patient could verbalize them.

Pharmaceutical companies understand a lot about the drugs they manufacture. But, just knowing the science (pharmacology) of a medication tells very little about any single patient's experience with it. Drug makers are scientists not physicians, and surely not patients. I don't know of any patient who ever started a drug company to make his/her own medicine. Do you?

Your physician "tries" medications on his/her patients based on teachings in medical school (long past and largely forgotten), the latest rap from visiting pharmaceutical reps, and the hype in the medical media. Sometimes, even from patients asking about such things as the Purple Pill. A tiny few physicians do individual study or go for continuing education on medications. But too often, such latter events turn out to be drug company paid vacations, promotions of pills and equipment, audiovisual slide extravaganzas, and/or medico-political rallies.

Consider now the dozens, hundreds or thousands of drugs available for physician "trials" and use. It would be quite an accomplishment for him/her to REALLY KNOW much about even a small number of those meds.

Oftentimes, the drug makers don't even really know as much as they should about the pills that they produce and push. The reader might pick up a Physicians' Desk Reference some day and peruse the technical sections regarding common drugs.

Actually, the PDR is hard to pick up these days. It used to be a few hundred pages long (400+ in 1950), but now it is contained in two bulky volumes, tight print, thin paper, 3000 pages, weighing more than 8 pounds. The PDR is the modern drug bible, consulted by practically all physicians, and sponsored (paid) by the drug companies which fill its print with information on well over 4000 pharmaceuticals.

An intent reader of the PDR will discover that the mechanisms of the supposed actions of most drugs are often incompletely understood. Even aspirin's effects are still not fully known. "More research into these therapeutic mechanisms are needed and under active consideration," is a typical conclusion for the data on any particular drug.

"Physicians prescribe . . . for diseases of which they know less."

You think, "At least, they understand my disease?"

On some occasions, they do. In most situations and with most conditions, they don't. (See In the Name of . . .)

Like drugs, there are more diseases in the modern era. Or at least, there seem to be. Because physicians and scientists have been discovering and identifying an endless list of syndromes, diseases, symptom-complexes, ills and ailments, affections, conditions, contagions, disorders, maladies, pathoses. And, that ain't all!

Hundreds of newly cataloged diseases seem to have called the growing number of medical specialties into being. Maybe it is the other way around. The growing number of specialists need more diseases to treat. Note: To discover a "new" disease is a real honor. It might be appropriate to interject here that specialties and specialization are not peculiar to medicine but to our whole modern society. Generalists like general practitioners are passe in the USA. I am told that GPs are still fairly common in the United Kingdom. There are certainly benefits from specialization, but just as certainly malign effects. Specialists lose track of The Big Picture and often don't even have a clue that one exists. People and their ills are really Big Picture issues.

Interestingly, there are few medical specialties devoted to specific diseases. In part because there are few specific diseases. We do have oncologists (specialists in cancer, of which there are dozens of types reminding us how little the disease is understood), rheumatologists, and infectious disease doctors. Rheumatology itself is a very non-specific specialty (another oxymoron) that tries to fill some gaps in medicine. You might be interested to consider the wide range of ills which rheumatology attempts to address.

Specialists generally work on PARTS of the BODY. Eye doctor, ENT, dentist, foot doctor, abdominal surgeon, chest cutter, psychiatrist (head man). Then, there are specialists for age groups: pediatricians and geriatricians. Women have their own specialty: gynecology.

You might think that the body has been covered by now with all these specialties and subspecialties. Not quite. The writer figures more specialties are on the way. One day, we may well have right eye doctors and left eye doctors. What do you think?

The author had thought the last idea was original. But while editing this book, he ran across the following quote in his extracurricular reading: "[Ancient Egyptians] had put everything to such a degree of specialization that we must conclude they had many centuries of civilization. There was a specialist for one eye and a specialist for the other, a specialist for the eyebrow, and so on. In my poor humble opinion, we are the Egyptians." (From a speech given by William Q. Judge in 1892, published in *Echoes of the Orient*, p. 524)

The simple fact that physicians have formed hundreds of specialties and categorized thousands of diseases clearly suggests that they are often "chasing ghosts."

"Physicians prescribe . . . to patients of which they know absolutely nothing."

Here is the most important part of the equation. We can address that concern very directly by asking you a few questions: How much does your physician or surgeon really know about you? How much can s/he learn in ten or fifteen minutes' time spent with you in a crowded schedule in a stuffy treatment room?

On the other hand, how much are you even willing to tell him? How able are you to put into words what is really going on in your body and in your life? What would it take for your doctor to fully interpret your experience, understand your discomfort, and know what is going on in your body, mind, life?

Well then, nobody's perfect. Neither physicians nor patients.

Physicians need patients and patients need physicians, but often for more than the usual suspect reasons. Thus, we continue on. Old patterns, same results.

When asked about my old profession, I used to tell acquaintances (but rarely patients): "I *practice* medicine." Interestingly, many people didn't get the idea at all. "Does that mean you're a doctor?" They had never heard that physicians *practice* medicine. Others got the meaning because of the inflection I put into the word *practice*.

If I told a patient, he might take it the wrong way and think maybe he had put himself in questionable hands. "I'm paying you real money. I want real medicine. Aren't you a real doctor not somebody who is just *practicing*?"

Sharing the idea on occasion with a friend was less problematic.

Doctors in fact *practice* medicine just like attorneys *practice* law. The work of both professions is very subjective. Medicine even more so than law.

"Standard medical *practice*" has many traditions, protocols and guidelines. Tests and procedures help point practitioners toward supposed workable diagnoses and labels. There are even algorithms (standardized steps used to solve problems) which can assist novices and assistants in following lines of investigation.

But in dealing with any individual patient, there is a huge spectrum of possibilities and questions to consider. Every body is different. Every person is also different. Likewise, every physician is different. A wise modern physician knows that. Does yours?

This is where the ART of medicine comes in. On more than a few occasions, I have thought it might be provocative and revealing for a TEST to be done of medicine and its practitioners. By taking a number of real patients with undiagnosed conditions and sending them to ten different physicians. Then comparing patterns of practice and treatments given by the providers. The survey being done with video would make for an interesting movie.

This sort of thing is rarely done in medicine. (Almost all medical exams, even board certifications, are done by written tests.) The exceptions seem to be in the context of training. Or when a physician is suspected of engaging in non-standard, questionable medical practices. The profession takes it on faith that Regular Physicians are "following standard *practice*" unless they hear otherwise from patients or peers.

I had my own small taste of such a video experience during my medical school training - third year. In one of our Family *Practice* programs, each of us was assigned a new patient to interview before a videotaping camera. The interview was then discussed in the presence of other students and a supervising physician. Each student was further expected to follow his/her patient over the course of the year.

Joyce was selected as my patient. I first met her only moments before the video interview. We sat rather uncomfortably before the camera as I conducted one of my first clinic interviews. Joyce and I had a wide-ranging conversation that allowed me to bring out things about her which had not been previously discovered.

Joyce was a thinnish, black woman in her late thirties who came to the Hospital Clinic in downtown Houston that day because of left-sided chest and arm pain. She had, just moments before, consulted with a Family *Practice* resident. That physician, who was already trained in psychiatry, had conducted a standard history and examination of the patient. He then ordered blood tests and a heart tracing. The procedures revealed "no significant abnormality." All that was and is quite standard procedure, but didn't do Joyce much good. It likely cost her more money than she could afford.

During our interview, I learned that Joyce had grown up in Louisiana and had moved to Houston some years ago with her husband and daughter. She was recently separated from him and didn't know his whereabouts. Her only daughter, aged seven years, was staying with Joyce's mother in Louisiana, partly for financial reasons. I never determined the other part. Joyce was quite alone and missed her daughter "too much." Still, she seemed to have some ambivalence about the situation.

Joyce thought her general health was "pretty good." She had, however, undergone a total hysterectomy some months previously for reasons which are now quite forgotten by me. Joyce showed little emotion during the interview, tearing but once when speaking of her daughter. She did admit to occasional moments of loneliness and depression. Joyce took no medication routinely and had not been offered estrogen replacement (standard *practice* at the time) when her ovaries were removed during her recent operation.

Joyce generally worked as a store clerk, but had recently moved to a new job. There it was. The obvious, outer cause of her chest pain. It had been entirely overlooked by the psychiatrist-turned-family practitioner in his undoubtedly brief and hurried moments with Joyce. You see, Joyce had only a few days previously taken on new work as an elevator operator in an old downtown office building. Joyce's job was relatively easy, taking people up and down the building levels. "Oh, I don't mind it. I kind of like it." Joyce merely had to conduct people, push buttons, and manually open and close the elevator door using her left arm. Open and close. Open and close with the left arm. Open and close.

The obvious cause of Joyce's chest pain was missed because the resident physician was concerned about and looking for a heart attack: rather unlikely though it was in a woman in her thirties. In Joyce's situation, a heart attack was unlikely, a muscle strain and pain due to relative overexertion was more common sensical. Joyce was not unusual, nor was her problem. Yet, she was a unique person who deserved more than a simple cookbook approach to a significant incident in her life.

There were deeper dimensions to her story which I didn't fully realize at the time. One dimension related to her hysterectomy and inability to bear more children. Joyce had suffered the loss of ovarian hormones and the disruption of function in her whole reproductive and endocrine system due to her surgery. More importantly, she was trying to deal with her separation from child and husband. All those factors were no doubt affecting her and must have contributed to her chest pain and "heart ache."

My contribution to Joyce's well-being was limited. I did get her started on estrogen replacement (standard *practice*). I saw her in the clinic and spoke to her over the telephone from time to time. I should have visited Joyce in her home surroundings. I did listen to her and encourage her attempts to improve communication with her daughter. I shared her life in a small way and for only a short time. But, hopefully, I did so in a humanistic and caring and somewhat artful manner.

Looking back over many years, I wonder whether a third-year medical student didn't have for a moment more of a sense of authentic medicine than a man completing his second residency. Regular Physicians often follow form and quickly go into testing mode. If a third-year novice can find a simpler, less expensive, and yet caring way to deal with patients, so too can fully trained physicians.

And, Mr. Voltaire would be the happier that physicians practiced another of his pithy quotes: "The art of medicine consists in amusing the patient while nature cures the disease."

Insuring Care?

Health Care and Health Insurance have many obvious connections as well as a subtler one. The latter being that they are both oxymorons.

Really? Really!

Let's start with Health Care: From the author's vantage point, there is no such thing as Health Care. How so?

Doctors don't really DO Health Care. They don't study health and they don't know what health is. Many would admit that to be the case. They might even say, "Health? Why, that's not my job. I work with people when they're sick. If you're interested in Health, go to the Wellness Center."

Since Wellness comes up, we might address that too. The Wellness movements are worthy and generally point in positive and hopeful, even healthful directions. "Small steps in the right direction," you might say.

But Wellness, like Prevention, is an unwanted stepchild of Father Medicine. Both get little in the way of attention, money and research in most medical circles.

Wellness programs rarely have much physician input, again because docs don't know much about it. Practically no one does. Besides, "Wellness doesn't pay Well." Para-professionals take on Wellness and do the best they can with limited resources and also limited knowledge. Physicians certainly don't want to be put out of business. Health and Wellness are not IN.

Most Wellness programs are hodge-podges of stress relief, exercise, nutrition, weight reduction, smoking cessation, and alternatives classes. There is rarely an over-riding Health philosophy to such programs.

True Health and Wellness efforts require some investment in Health philosophy. Wholeness as another name for Health touches on matters of spirit and religion which are other areas of which materialistic "workers in disease" must beware.

Physicians really don't CARE for your HEALTH. They are in Disease Care mode and focused almost exclusively on disease. Generally speaking, the few efforts made in a medical office towards Health are left in the hands of nurses and assistants, literature and video material.

Health to many Regular Physicians remains "the absence of disease." They weren't trained about Health - and still aren't. Even if they had been, they would have rebelled against it. "Health class? The profs are taking us back to high school days," I'm sure medical students would say.

The closest med students get to Health is in Physiology class where the body is "broken" apart into systems. Physicians-to-be learn about normal function of body parts and systems. They can tell you about blood counts, arterial pressures, urine outputs, respiratory rates, and the like. Both normal and abnormal. But, Health for a whole being is not addressed. This is one of the Big Gaps in medicine, past and present.

Generally speaking, medical training and medical students are focused on the "meat and potatoes" medicine which equates to pathology and disease, blood and guts, cutting and curing, saving lives. Not "salad and vegetables," like prevention and health oriented topics.

This reminds the writer of his days taking Basic Sciences in med school. The curriculum called for a number of hours in Computer

Sciences. Can you imagine such a thing?! John Lenahan, Ph.D., led us in a few hours of classroom studies involving computer applications along with some lab exercises meant to teach us rudiments of computer programming. A very modest introduction to the subject.

You should have heard the grumbling. "What has this got to do with medicine? We will never use this stuff." How little did they know - any of us know - how important computers would become in modern life, including medicine, in the coming years. Health is/was surely an even more important topic for medics, but one for which there was not a single class provided.

True Health is a Big Picture thing which requires people - physicians or patients - to look beyond illness and problems and the body. It takes time and a different orientation.

YOU don't go to the doctor's office when you are healthy, generally. The vast portion of medical visits are for illness and injury or followup appointments. Healthy people don't take the time to see their practitioner except for annual physical exams and vaccinations. Many people don't even do that.

So in a sense, YOU are part of the problem. Unless YOU take Health seriously. Then, maybe you really don't need to spend much time at all with our present Disease Care system.

Disease Care prevails because of our general mindset, because physicians have disease on the brain, and because fear rules in society and in medicine. The road from Disease Care to Health Care will surely be a long one.

~~~~~~

The other side of the coin - and this chapter - is Health Insurance. Which is also an oxymoron and presents similar ideas for consideration by thoughtful, frugal and prudent people.

The Industrial Era has brought us to a period where we are controlled by our imagined futures. Business and commerce have been forced to prepare for our retirements and illnesses. Forget health. Aging and disease and death are of supreme importance.

Thus, millions and millions plan their lives around so-called health insurance, IRAs, investment portfolios. "I must have it all planned out before I leave my job and retire." "My Roth IRA is a slam dunk to take care of my future needs." "I can't change jobs unless the new one has health insurance." "The job isn't important, even if I hate it. It's the benefits."

The media is forever reminding us that Social Security is inadequate and no one has enough insurance. For the richest country in the world to have "so little" seems ironic and paradoxical. How much is enough?

No one seems to earn enough (have you ever met anyone who willingly admits to earning more money than s/he needs?), and most everyone spends too much. And while we all get sick and die, most of us think the doctor and the hospital have magic bullets to save us from pain and delay the inevitable.

We have bought into the idea of retirement packages, financial planning, and health insurance like other withering fairy tales akin to Happily Ever After. Hollywood, Wall Street and the Mayo Clinic mentality have led us down the path towards a supposed unending bed of roses. While the Western systems have held up remarkably well for many decades, it is clear that many of those systems are near the breaking point.

Stock brokers will admit that their business is all based on paper. No common stock has any intrinsic value. Insurance policies are promises to pay. Promises are not always kept. Pensions are not always honored as written. We see that in the present day. Likewise, insurance packages are simply not what they are touted to be.

Health Insurance is akin to Life Insurance. They both sound good, positive and wholesome. But, they are both deceptive. Life Insurance is clearly Death Insurance. What about Health Insurance? You got it. It is most assuredly Disease Insurance.

The simple fact is that HEALTH INSURANCE does not exist! Neither insurance nor the greatest physician in the world can assure your health. People fall over dead the day after getting a clean bill of health from their doctors.

More physicians and more medicine will never assure your health. Sometimes they can help, but they may also do more harm than good. You might just reflect for a moment on the general states of health of medical professionals. They are not a particularly healthy lot and succumb to all sorts of diseases, addictions, suicides.

We get used to things as they are and often don't notice that "A spade is not always a spade." Health insurance is surely a misnomer. It is simply Disease Insurance. It insures that when you feel bad, get sick and think you need a doctor, you will be able to use his/her services without paying the whole bill for all the appointments and tests and procedures which result when you consult your physician.

Your Disease Insurance does a number of things, some of which you most likely have never considered.

- Disease Insurance promotes using the medical system and, in fact, grows the system. "Ah, I got insurance. I have two policies. It won't cost me a nickel to spend a few minutes with the doctor."

Insured patients prompt physicians to order more tests, probe to the extent of coverage, and make full use of insurance. Self-payers think twice before venturing into the system. They save money and lower patient volume at medical offices.

- As the system has expanded and grown, all sorts of things have crept into "standard practice." Like more paperwork, more paper workers, more intrusion by insurance companies. Standardized care has replaced personal care to a large degree.

Third parties, like Disease Insurance companies and Medicare and Medicaid, also make more and more medical decisions. That is so regardless of what kind of physician you consult.

- Disease Insurance supports more testing and operative procedures. Certain diagnoses mandate certain patterns of testing. Insurance companies have to protect themselves (CYA), just like Regular Physicians. Medical insurance has much in common with malpractice insurance. They both are intent on protecting against the worst, however unlikely such may be.

Thus the volume of procedures increases as do the number of them available for your physician to choose from. The whole mentality proceeds to growth and duplication and re-duplication of testing. Many tests are repeated needlessly and wastefully. Charts get voluminous and report files get thick. Often with little valuable information rising out of the mass of paperwork and technology.

AND, you guessed it. All this activity adds to costs to the patient and, directly or indirectly, to increased physician income.

- The Disease Insurance that many people are proud to own actually empowers the concept of disease and supports the disease model of modern medicine. Insurance enables physicians to search for and find more diseases, ailments and conditions to treat.

A large proportion of those conditions may not warrant treatment. Another portion may be made worse by intervention. (The treatment may be worse than the disease.) And then, there are the ill effects which are common in therapy of all sorts of problems. Even a sugar pill can have side effects.

- Disease Insurance adds to the medicalization of life, spreading tentacles hither thither and yon. Medicine and testing thus become required to apply for many jobs, to play little league baseball, to get married, etc. Medicine intrudes everywhere and in so doing finds as well as creates more disease.

Disease hunts become increasingly common. Diabetes gets promoted through Diabetes Month. Depression gets a nod through Depression Screening Tests. Another telethon is begun, another benefit produced. Disease is not lessened, but really increased.

A Frugal Physician is aware of the contradictions implicit in words like Health Care and Health Insurance and so should you be. Disease Care is necessary, but tell it like it is. Do the same with Disease Insurance until Health becomes key in medical practice.

Bizness

Medicine has become business - Big Business. The medical system is overgrown, super-specialized, hyper-technical, papered over and out of control in many ways. Reform is in the air. Legislation - to "fix" the system - which has been debated for decades, has been passed at the federal level in the USA.

But Federal intervention is likely to have little real effect on the expensive state of medical care, much of which is ineffective and off target. At the rate things are going, we will continue to have more medical care, more technology, more bureaucracy, and more insurance of one kind or another.

More medical care (disease care) - more of the same - is hardly the solution. Science and technology have brought us into an era of problems in medicine akin to ones in our military system. Surely, it is better to put money into hospitals and medical technology than into guns and weapons. But, neither seems to be particularly effective in dealing with modern society and its real challenges. They both have been promulgated out of fear and add to massive waste in our modern life.

More than fifty years ago, President Eisenhower warned of a developing Military-Industrial Complex. He saw it coming and the first MIC has long since become part of our everyday world. Bigger weapons - including nuclear warheads and missiles - were supposed to protect us and keep us safe. But, they may have done the opposite. Business interests have steered a great deal of policy with regard to national defense and military power, war regalia and weapons procurement.

Now, similar forces have brought us MIC II: the Medical-Industrial Complex. The general thinking is like, "We have protected the nation and the whole Western world with missiles, fighter jets, and modern technology. We can create comparable wonders in clinics and hospitals with smaller doses of Big Tech."

In actual fact, medicine hasn't kept up - with or without technologies

- with many other sciences. As a society, we might question: "Have the trillions of dollars spent in medical care and research in recent decades paid off?" "When was the last time, we heard of a 'real cure?'" "Have all those million-dollar scanning devices - CT, MRI, PET - made substantial differences in quality of life for those who spend big money on them?" "Has the extension in lifespan of J Q Public brought more health or just more years?"

The wonders of modern medicine are too often ones which leave individuals wondering: "What did I get out of all of those tests?" "Why did I let them put me through all of that rigamarole?" "Just one more procedure. Then, one more. How many more can there be?" "What did I pay those thousands of dollars for? I have the same problems plus financial ones now."

Medical technology has helped bring about the huge expansion in medical business. Every level of the profession is affected. And this force has rolled on into almost every aspect of our lives.

The changes are most obvious in big clinics and hospitals. But, they affect - maybe infect - the smallest of medical operations.

• For practical purposes, the old time GP is history in the USA. S/he has been replaced by Family Practitioners who are supposed to be generalists. These FPs are intended to be the modern version of yesterday's General Practitioners.

But curiously in these days, a generalist becomes specialized - board certified in Family Practice. That sure seems like another oxymoron to me. What do you think?

• The general effect of this state of medicine is for Family Practitioners to only treat patients with very simple problems. And others that have become chronic. Those which the specialists pass back to the Referring Physicians.

Still, Referring Physicians are theoretically important to the system because they keep patients in the pipeline to the real specialists. But more and more, consumers make their own referrals and try to bypass physicians at the lower echelons of care. They think, "Why should I waste time and money with Dr. Doe, when I know he is going to refer me up the line, anyway?"

The old time doctor just has a tough time keeping a toehold because of the flow of the modern medical system. Exceptions are in remote and rural areas and where conscious physicians make choices to do things differently, regardless of consequences with the looming system.

It is harder for most solo practitioners. They have to compete for patients. They have to do things just like the big boys and clinics, order and refer, order and refer. It is harder and harder for imagination and compassion to find room in the system.

When patients start having more imagination of their own, they will help the situation by seeking providers who have imagination as well as common sense, compassion and competence.

• Few simple remedies are used anymore. Poultices, rubdowns, sponge baths, salt packs and the like are almost ancient history. "Why should we do things manually when we can do them with machines and medications? Medications have been manufactured to the highest standards of quality. A person can not be sure what goes into those herbal preparations. They are not purified and refined like pharmaceuticals. I dare not recommend such things!"

Old time, hands-on treatments are out, in part, because their value is hard to prove. Numbers and statistics and paperwork rule. Still, real proof is not to be had either with standard practice or with alternatives. And human contact and touch are becoming as nought. Or almost so.

• Technology is king. There is a test or procedure, or battery of them, for practically every ailment. And, they certainly must be used. "Because that is the modern standard. This is the twenty-first century. No ailment need go untested."

"Bigger is better," so we have been told. But, we are beginning to recognize that ain't necessarily so. The new methods are meant to improve things. But, then there is less and less time for face-to-face contact with patients. "Yes, but there is a waiting line. Anyway, we go by results. And if not results, by numbers."

- Speed is of the essence. That is part of the reason we have Air Ambulance programs. Helicopter evacuations were developed in war zones for serious casualties with no other transportation access to get prompt care.

  These days, such services are grossly overused and dramatically increase medical costs. How many times have I seen helicopters pick up patients who could have been transported just as easily by ground ambulance! Sometimes, more quickly.

  This common situation was brought home to me as I saw a rancher friend drawn through the "faster is better" medical system. This middle-aged man had been thrown from his horse while he was moving cattle one spring. John got back on his horse and continued down the trail for most of an hour. Eventually, the hardened herdsman was in so much pain that he asked to be driven into the hospital which was about seventy miles away.

  A friend did the duty, but stopped at a small town twenty miles en route. Before a person could turn around, EMTs were collecting, administering oxygen, placing a neck brace on him, and putting him on a hard backboard. (standard protocol) Instead of driving him the rest of the way into the medical center, someone decided a helicopter ambulance was needed.

  It took much longer to get him moved by ambulance - to a landing area and then helicoptered 45 miles to the medical center than it would have to simply take him direct by ground ambulance. Two hours had passed since the incident occurred. (Interestingly, the latter vehicle is called a Quick Response Unit.) John's travel bill was certainly increased tenfold. He was found to have a lacerated kidney which resolved on its own. His body took care of the problem while he was tested for several days in the hospital.

- The modern medical business feeds on itself. Offices require larger staffs. Overhead goes up. More patients are required or patients pay more because office bills expand. Or both.

  Hospitals have so much expensive equipment which soon becomes outdated, have to meet the highest building codes, and compete with neighboring facilities to be the best in the region.

- Medicine, furthermore, is monopolistic. The modern medical monopoly makes the system monolithic and hard to change (it is actually duolithic - drugs and surgery). Almost all questions of health and disease are decided within the confines of an inbred system which has little external input, attention or control.

Peer Review supposedly governs medical work and issues. But, physicians rarely bother each other in their work. Certainly, non-physicians - excepting legislators and insurance companies - have practically no say in major medical concerns. Malpractice and non-standard practice and drug abuse are notable exceptions.

- Consumers have no say regarding the costs of their medical care. Too often they don't have an inkling what their bill will look like until they see it in the mail. Costs and bills thus can't help but rise.

Your Regular Physician is a businessman whether s/he admits it or not. But, s/he has absolutely no training in business. Physicians are notoriously bad business people. They weren't helped at all by their training which likely never had an hour devoted to medical business, costs of services, and patients' generally unspoken need to have their finances considered as part of their state of health.

The "business of medicine" has large implications. A Frugal Physician makes it his/her business to ask about patients' financial situations. True health surely encompasses a host of forces.

In the future, the business of medicine inevitably will be more about:
- people than paperwork
- persons and not just bodies
- patients and not merely diseases or cases
- simplicity rather than complexity
- comfort and compassion ahead of diagnosis and treatment
- the whole person including his/her wallet
- the profession of healing

Working in Pain

Clinics and hospitals are extraordinary places to work as well as do business. Transactions are hardly ever simple and straightforward like those which consumers make at the grocery or hardware, laundry or restaurant.

Every business has a psychological component which is often the most difficult part of making a concern successful. But, medical businesses have Psychology written all over them.

There are so many facets of medical practice and business which even a clairvoyant would be taxed to gather in and assess. Most of them are psycho-social-spiritual in nature. Little do most physicians and patients realize that situation as they focus on the physical body and look for disease.

Of course, one could speak similarly about life in general. That would hit the nail on the head. But as medicine regularly deals with pain and fear, disease and injury, life and death issues, the intensity of inner issues can be tremendous. If only we could get glimpses of the subtle forces that focus through the drama of birth, the agony of trauma and injury, the impact of sudden illness, the weight of chronic disease, the heartache of psychotic episodes, the impotence at the death bed.

But then again, maybe we can. Maybe we have. If we can imagine it, then it can be so.

Pain is of central importance in the medical setting. It is always more than skin deep, so to speak. Pain affects providers as well as patients, whether they realize it or not.

I have had a number of medical friends over the years who "took on pain" in somewhat extraordinary ways. Cindy started a pain clinic in association with an anesthesiologist. She did counseling and biofeedback and the like. It suited her personality in some ways and the clinic attracted a substantial clientele. It became a "good" business.

Well, good enough. But, Cindy had her own aches and discomforts. To top it all off, she used to tell people who asked her what she did for a living, "I work in pain."

Most people wouldn't have paid an extra moment's notice on that comment. But I sure did. So, Cindy might have if she had paid attention to her own words.

Another friend worked her way into a New York City pain management clinic. Gina went from little income to $60,000 a year working as a massage therapist and unit supervisor. She got to work with physicians and therapists in an orthodox setting. Something Gina had dreamed about for years.

"Working in pain," however, she took on patient's problems physically, emotionally and probably otherwise. Being a very sensitive person, Gina often carried her work home with her.

There were layers to the pain she was dealing with. Helping others can help heal ourselves, but that is not always the case.

Gina already carried her own aches and pains from childhood and married years. Then, she lived in one of the most crowded and congested cities in the world. Surrounded by all sorts of negative and even malign energies, Gina was susceptible to more of their influence than she ever knew.

Those were just the first few layers. Then, she went to work in a big hospital filled with stressed and sick, ill and injured people. Not all of them were patients.

Furthermore, she took on a "job in pain." She got close to people, touched them, heard their stories over and over. That could be tough on the hardiest soul. Talk about Intensity. "Working in pain" in a busy hospital in one of the largest cities in the world.

"Well, somebody has to do it," you might say. Maybe so, but Gina didn't have to. Fortunately, her physician employer saw the writing on the wall and gently eased her out the door. Eventually to other less stressful work.

We can neither avoid pain nor loss in life. Pain is one of those slippery symptoms that medicine has so much trouble grasping and quantitating. Medicine tries to quantitate everything. Physicians haven't found useful ways to quantify pain. They are still trying. In the meantime, they try to "manage" this potent yet elusive nemesis.

I had my own brief exposure to the world of "pain management" during the last year of my medical school career. That fourth year was almost all electives, many of which I took outside of the Texas Medical Center. I then charted my course in areas of medicine which were as humanistic and holistic as possible. I heard about an elective in Pain Management, thought "That sounds unusual, maybe innovative," and signed up. I really didn't know what I was getting into until I showed up for duty.

The program put me back in the Hermann Hospital for a month with a fair amount of my time passed in the Operating Suite. But, the circumstances were quite a bit different from earlier days. A resident in Maxillofacial Surgery and I spent a month working under Dr. Claude Duval, a French-Canadian anesthesiologist turned pain specialist.

Dr. Duval treated patients with intransigent pain by using various types of anesthetic procedures. When common methods for pain relief were found lacking, patient failures were sent on to Dr. Duval. For the most part, Duval used paraspinal blocks in attempts to deaden or quiet irritated, inflamed, or uncooperative nerves. The blocks were intended to break the pain cycle of suffering patients. A large group of his patients had failed herniated disk surgeries. There were some obvious defects in Duval's theory, but patients kept being referred and Dr. Duval was only too pleased to keep treating them.

I remember one particular patient, George Willing, who had been operated and re-operated FIVE times for low back pain and diagnosed herniated disk. George was a spunky and affable little fellow despite all his misfortune. I think the surgeries had cut him down an inch or two in size. He listed to one side, had a foot drop, and could only walk short distances without great difficulty. Mr. Willing spent most of his time in bed or in a wheelchair. We treated George on a number of occasions with paraspinal blocks to try to short-circuit his pain syndrome.

Performing a paraspinal block was a good way to keep three or four medical personnel busy for a couple hours. The procedure was posted on the OR schedule and we set up a tiny OR suite with the necessary materials. Dr. Duval supervised the whole procedure, yet was able to circle the department looking in on other cases.

Placed in a prone position (face down) on an OR table, the sedated patient only received light anesthetic gas while we plunged six large bore 12-inch long needles into his paraspinal muscles. The objective was to place the ends of the needles (three on each side of the spine) close to the paraspinal sympathetic ganglia. We shot portable Xrays to "eyeball" our rather blind efforts. Dr. Duval reviewed the films and made judgments about needle placement. Quite frequently, we had us extract a needle or two for reinsertion. I never figured out Dr. Duval's criteria for determining the accuracy of placement. When the needles were acceptably lined up, we slowly injected 50 cc (about 2 ounces) of a Novocaine-like solution via each needle into the paraspinal muscle mass.

Whenever we took George through this procedure, he had immediate pain relief lasting for 24 to 48 hours. He would be ready to leave the hospital, when he developed an abnormal heart rhythm. George was then transferred to the coronary care unit for observation for several hours. The internists wisely abstained from undertaking any major intervention during those interludes. Soon, he was back on the ward with a normal heart rate and rhythm, but his back pain returned as well. The cycle was complete, but a new one would be initiated before long with another round of short-lived, symptomatic pain relief. Somewhere along the line, George took the hint and quietly slipped out of the hands of the Pain Management team. He was not seen again, at least while I was around.

Ben Davis was an even more memorable patient admitted to the Pain Service. Ben, his wife, Emily, and I developed a comfortable rapport, almost a friendship, and maintained a communication for many months. Davis was a semi-retired oil and gas leasing agent who had prided himself on his fitness and activity. He was referred to Dr. Duval because of chronic, excruciating pain in his right groin. The pain was originally thought to be caused by an inguinal hernia which was routinely repaired several months before he appeared at the Hermann Hospital. By the time Ben reached the Pain Service, he had been through quite a medical ordeal already and his travails were only just beginning.

In hopes that the cause of his pain might be discovered and some relief afforded, Ben had submitted to numerous surgical procedures following on the heels of his hernia repair. His first operative site was explored and a synthetic patch was implanted there - for what purpose I could never determine. On another occasion, his belly was explored and, finding nothing of great consequence, the surgeon excised Ben's appendix so as not to return from his expedition empty handed. On a further visit to the OR, the patch was removed and the original incision re-approximated. Shortly before coming to the University Hospital, Ben had met with a neurosurgeon who was reticent to intervene in his complicated and perplexing case. That physician did no more than suggest the use of a TNS (Transcutaneous Neuro Stimulator) and recommend a visit with Dr. Duval. Duval readily took on his case and sold Ben on the potential for real benefit from a series of paraspinal blocks.

I was delegated the task of doing Ben's admitting history and physical examination. He and I went over the usual medical territory and then settled down to a good visit and got to know each other a bit. Only as his hospitalization progressed did I get to know Mrs. Davis. Later, Emily corresponded with me and kept me abreast of her husband's tortuous and torturous medical travels.

Ben was a feisty Texan with a dose of vinegar in his belly and a sparkle in his eye. He was in his mid-sixties, but by no means ready to kick back. He had "too much life to live." Ben also had high hopes - too high - that Dr. Duval's method would give him real relief. So did Dr. Duval. By that time, I was getting pretty skeptical of the whole process on the Pain Service. I had seen nothing to suggest to me that any of the procedures performed did more than cover up pain for a few hours to a few days, weeks at the most.

Ben's turn arrived and we went through the paraspinal block routine with the six giant needles, the portable Xray check for placement, and the anesthetic injections. As expected, there was a rapid and dramatic decrease in pain. Ben had none - for a short time - and he was pleased, almost excited. He got out of bed at the first chance, walked and smiled while anticipating the best.

Alas! The relief was transient. Within forty-eight hours, Ben's pain was back with a vengeance. Davis experienced both mental and physical agony. He told me, "I must get back to my life. I tell you I'm going to beat this damn pain - or die in the attempt. I can't live with this pain."

We repeated the procedure two more times. Ben and Dr. Duval still hoped for some lasting results. They were not forthcoming. After the third round, Ben went home, a small town a couple hours northeast of Houston, to consider his options. He left with his pain masked only slightly by the TNS, but no regrets for his fruitless experiences at the Texas Medical Center. His hopes were dampened, but not drowned. Davis did not give up easily. Mrs. Davis held his hand when he let her and sent me letters from time to time about Ben's continuing medical engagements.

Pain is one of those often inexplicable, very subjective and clearly personal experiences in life. Physician attempts to elicit useful information about the nature of pain are commonly futile. Their inevitable testing and procedures are based on weak initial information, narrow physical approaches to the problem, and ungainly attempts at intervention.

A Frugal Physician avoids jumping to conclusions and starting medical processes that can get out of hand. S/he tempers the fears which swirl around patients in pain and tries to let common sense and natural forces do their work even when discomforting. S/he knows that intervention too often makes things worse.

S/he also knows, "Pain is inevitable. Suffering is optional."

Fear Not

Like many medical professionals, Cindy (see previous chapter) had her own issues as well as skills which made the pain clinic the right place for her to be. At least for a time. She eventually moved on to another profession.

Before I met her, she had expended some extra money and bought a bright, shiny red Mitsubishi sports car. Now, it is general knowledge that RED stands out from the background most any place. Just as much on the highway.

Cindy took her new red car out on the highway, let her hair loose, and pushed her foot down on the accelerator. Probably more than a few times.

It wasn't long before she caught a Highway Patrolman's attention. Then, he got her attention and gave her an ample-sized speeding ticket.

Another picture of Cindy leads to a punch line. One day, we went for a drive in my car. From the passenger seat, Cindy cleared her throat and said, "Robert, do you have any defects?"

It didn't take me long to respond, "You mean like being critical and fault-finding. Yeah, I have those and a few more."

She didn't say anything for some time, so I figured it was her turn to answer the question, "How about you, Cindy. Do you have any defects?"

It took her a couple moments to answer while I turned my head in her direction. Cindy raised her nose into the air, pointed her finger and said disgustedly, "Well, I get a hair that grows out of my chin every once in a while. And I have to pluck it out. Ooh!"

That may have been a Big Defect for a counselor in those days.

I'm not sure about the present state of counseling.

But, Cindy had others including a quite obvious one to those with eyes to see. She had broadcast it to the whole world when she bought her new car and applied for a personalized license plate. If the color of her new vehicle didn't get the Highway Patrolman's attention, her plate should have. It got mine.

Cindy's plate read FEARNOT. If there had been room (only seven letters allowed) it might more correctly have read FEAR NOT? Cindy, her patients and all patients have FEAR as a common part of their life experience and presenting medical problems.

Fear brings people to the doctor. No doubt about it. Fear of disease and pain open the gates to the medical system routines and subsequent outcomes.

Most patients appear in front of their physicians firstly because of discomfort in their lives and secondarily bodily illness. Often, they are quite unaware of the influences of the former on the latter. It is easy to focus on the body, worry and fret about it. Which readily takes one's mind off the "bigger issues."

Some patients are just feeling bad and want to feel better. But, a high percentage are afraid something serious or deadly is going to happen to them. Our medical system and the mainstream media often add to our common worries.

Lord Salisbury, three times prime minister of the United Kingdom, put medical worries into a big picture, "No lesson seems to be so deeply inculcated by the experience of life as that you should never trust experts. If you believe the doctors, nothing is wholesome: if you believe the theologians, nothing is innocent: if you believe the soldiers, nothing is safe."

FEAR is key. Fear causes us to do a lot of things. Fear certainly gets people to the doctor's office, clinic and emergency room. Sometimes, rightly so. Others, unnecessarily so because common sense is overwhelmed by other forces. Your physician often adds his/her share into the mix when you are scared and fretting. That seems to be an occupational hazard. Remember, doctors believe "nothing is wholesome" and are constantly looking for disease.

Seven major fears bring people to doctors for care:

1) Blemishes and bumps, rashes and itches get people's attention, especially when they're visible so that others can see them. While patients generally don't worry that their "skin will disintegrate," they

still don't want to be marked for the world to see their "leprous spots."

Dermatologists get rich on rashes. But, the vast majority of skin problems go away with or without their creams and lotions. Furthermore, there are almost no fatal skin diseases.

It should be apparent to most anybody, including physicians, that there are surely psychological aspects to every skin problem. Before, during and/or after onset.

In my military medical days, I saw a host of young people with skin problems. Rather than medicate them, I often gave them reassurance and referrals to the base dermatologist. I knew that a large percentage of their problems would disappear by the time their 90-day wait to see the Skin Doctor passed.

2) Problems with "private parts" are high on the list of common patient worries, especially in the younger age group. Urologists and gynecologists have many of the same sort of issues to deal with as skin doctors. A high percentage of their patients are scared about what is "growing in my groin."

It can certainly be distressing: "This is terrible, doc. I'm afraid it might fall off if it gets any worse." Sexually Transmitted Disease (STD) is quite common, but so too are simple skin blemishes that set up shop between the legs.

In the military, the urology clinic schedule was only a little less backed up than the derm department's. When referring, I knew that most soldiers given urology appointments, like dermatology patients, would be feeling better by the time their appointment came up some weeks or months later.

3) Problems with memory and thinking processes, seizures and dizzy spells are cause for great worry. "Doc, I think I'm losing my mind. Can you help me find it?"

No one is comfortable, if s/he thinks his/her mental apparatus is not working as usual. Yet, most of us will experience a variety of such symptoms. Especially as we grow older. Most complaints, however scary, pass away on their own - with or without treatment.

All of us will have some such spells in the course of our lives. On the other hand, if you develop a "real" neurological problem, "real" help from the medical profession is unlikely. The brain and spinal cord are still largely *terra incognita*. Even in the 21st century, neurologists and neurosurgeons still work relatively BLINDLY on most of their patients. But, that doesn't keep them from doing uncountable scans and Xrays and invasive procedures which rarely provide usable information or beneficial therapy.

A quote by neurologist Raymond Adams on the disease called epilepsy and its relationship to the nervous system may give the reader a sense of the wonder that still surrounds the brain and nerves in the present era. "Many physicians will find it curious, indeed almost comic, that neurology should be concerned with the treatment of an important entity (epilepsy) when it has little or no idea of its cause. The plain fact is that the very nature of the nervous system and this particular manifestation of nervous disease have defied analysis." (*Harrison's Principles of Internal Medicine*)

4) Chest pains and "heartaches" are also cause for big concern and understandably so. At least if you are not ready to die. When the heart seems to act up and the chest throbs, we worry about the BIG ONE. Yet, most such symptoms are not related to heart function.

While medical technology has lots of tests and protocols to deal with heart problems, the final verdict is not in on most of them. Many such procedures were never passed through reviews which medications have to undergo with the FDA. Bypasses, angioplasties, and stent placements are done routinely these days, but their benefits are almost totally unproven. Their costs are exorbitant.

5) Plain old pain, severe and unremitting, in any body part is likely to scare anyone and get the hardiest into a medical practitioner. Pain certainly can be a valuable tip as well as a warning sign.

But, what is it trying to tell us? This is an important question which too often goes unasked. C.S. Lewis may have had part of the answer when he said, "God whispers to us in our pleasures, speaks in our conscience, but shouts in our pain."

How many people listen? Really listen? Will you listen? Will your doctor?

6) The BIGGEST WORRY which gets people to their doctor is simply the fear of death, which hides behind some of the other fears. You might want to think that your physician can help you and prevent premature death, but physicians die just like their patients. Sometimes, at earlier ages.

We all must face our mortality. Rarely do physicians have power over life and death, and then only when delegated to them from Higher Hands. But, this is one place where a physician can be of help if s/he pays attention and really listens, and patients are willing to express their real fears.

7) Run-of-the-mill anxiety brings 'em in, maybe more than any thing else. Some patients are willing to admit, "My nerves are on edge. I get panic attacks. I can't go out into crowds."

However, many people's anxiety gets transformed into stomach upset, headaches, insomnia, sinus congestion, allergies, and hay fever. The list is very long. Many of these complaints are easily missed as being simply somatic (bodily) ailments.

Practically all of us would rather have problems in our bodies than in our minds. Physicians prefer it that way, too.

One of the major works of a physician is to allay anxiety. Not by the indirect route of passing time through the ordering tests or prescribing Valium. But, by getting to know the patient. Finding out what REALLY brought him/her to the office. Searching for what lies beneath the blemish, the discomfort, the pain, the ache. A Frugal Physician is just as concerned about your fears about your ailment, as about the condition itself. It likely will take more than 15 minutes to help you with them, but it will be worth it.

Hoofbeats

Not long after I parted from Dr. Kirkendall, the Hermann Hospital, and UTMSH, I began training in Family Practice at Martin Army Hospital in Fort Benning, Georgia. I walked the halls and made rounds with my fellow intern, Dr. Ed Friedler, on the Internal Medicine Service for two months. Practically every day, Ed would have a story to tell trying to support some point he wanted to make.

Interestingly, Winnie the Pooh, the Bear of Little Brain, was one of his main authorities. Long before the publication of the Tao of Pooh and similar books, Ed sang the praises of Pooh and quoted him frequently. Having never read or been read Winnie the Pooh books, I got a bit of an education regarding children's literature in the midst of my medical training. Thanks again, Ed.

And thanks for the painting and books you gave me on my 30th birthday. I received two Pooh books and a childlike but original painting of the Pooh characters by Friedler entitled "Consider All the Possibilities." That was one of Friedler's mottoes and became one of my own. But, we each created different layers of meaning for that particular slogan.

In a similar vein, Ed's most common refrain was one drawn from "western lore." He would regularly remind me, "Now Bob, what do we look for when we hear hoofbeats off in the distance?"

You might suspect that the answer was not the obvious one: "Horses." Ed's reminder and a recurring one in modern medicine is to "Look for zebras when you hear hoofbeats in the distance."

A physician - especially a novice - is supposed to consider ALL the possibilities. That causes him/her to often focus on some of the least likely in medical practice.

Really? Dr. Ed was making a sarcastic but pertinent remark about how we young investigating physicians had to spend so much time chasing after the unusual and scouring for the unique. Too often, Ed and I were ordering tests in the search of exotic diseases rather than tending to what seemed most obvious or at least likely. The pattern, which was around in the 70s, is just as common or more so in the present day.

Following on the last chapter, we might want to remember how pervasive anxiety and fear are. Whatever the diagnosis, fear and anxiety and emotions are always involved. I don't remember these being prominent possibilities in our list of differential diagnoses.

Nor do I recall ever having a medical school lecture on how anxiety affects patients, precipitates illness, gets them to doctors, magnifies their problems. It seems as in many problems, anxiety was separated out as an individual psychiatric disorder with many pseudonyms which elicited prescription for anti-anxiety drugs.

Medical school focused on big disease, the "real" stuff like pheochromocytoma. We were repeatedly lectured on the disease called pheochromocytoma in one course after another. Pheochromocytoma, a mouthful of a word and a rare disease - specific tumor of adrenal gland tissue - is one with marked symptoms and laboratory findings. We heard so much about pheochromocytoma because it is a dramatic disease and one of the few which is neatly diagnosed and readily treated with surgery.

But, most ailments are not simple, direct, and dramatic like pheochromocytoma. Here are some common examples that you might experience:

• If you go in for a checkup because you have aches and pains around your joints, you are likely to be tested and re-tested for rheumatoid arthritis.

Why? Because that kind of arthritis can be diagnosed with laboratory tests. Osteoarthritis is many times more common, but it's not easily diagnosed. There is no quick test for it. Xrays are often done, but are generally "equivocal" and wasteful. Still, most of us will experience some of the creaks and groans, aches and pains of aging which physicians like to call osteoarthritis.

• My brother often asks for medical advice but rarely takes it. I once complained to my sister-in-law, who said, "Don't feel bad. He doesn't follow the advice he pays for."

My sister-in-law called me about 2:00 am, some months ago. Brother had just tried to get out of bed. His head was spinning and he thought he was going to die. I didn't talk to him directly, but passed on that I had similar symptoms during the previous flu season. A neighbor had the full blown flu and vertigo as well. I just laid low until it passed in a few days. I don't know what the neighbor did.

I tried to suggest to my brother - through his wife - that he let the symptoms pass. But the next morning, he made an appointment with the Veterans Administration Center near his home. He got in quickly and was told he may have had a stroke. Then, he was passed through an expensive (for the government) set of scans. Those tests showed no pathology. "You may be getting Meniere's disease. Regardless, we probably should get you seen by a cardiologist."

- Cardiologists are plenty busy these days because simple chest discomfort, which can be caused by dozens of things, immediately produces the need for "a cardiogram and some blood tests." Then, there follow further studies looking for signs of a heart attack, blocked vessels, etc.

Yet, the chances of heart attack are low. Medical treatments for heart attack are questionable, unproven, and expensive. They commonly lead to dangerous, invasive procedures. The frequent use of Coumadin, a blood thinner originally used as rat poison, is fraught with complications. A very large percentage of patients using Coumadin will eventually have bleeding from one orifice or another. Beware!

Not long ago, a heart attack patient used to spend six weeks in the hospital for a simple myocardial infarction. Now, a few days or hours. In other countries, not at all. Many are sent home from the emergency room. Have patients changed - or medical practice?

Still, the punch line is that most chest problems are not even caused by the heart. How about the chest wall, spine, lungs, stomach, gall bladder. And points distant. Every thing is connected. And so are the emotions. How many people do you know who experienced "heartache" which caused them to get medical attention?

A middle-aged friend was attempting to be a schoolteacher for 30 fifth graders after a divorce and seeing her own children mostly grown. Between school stress, family concerns and being a sensitive soul, she started having "waves of overwhelm" focused in her chest. Ms. Grant took herself to the clinic. An EKG and other tests were ordered immediately. All were negative, but she had a decent sized bill and suggestions for further scans. Fortunately, Ms. Grant tuned into some of the clues and realized how she was unconsciously focusing her problems in her chest.

- "Those skin lesions may be cancerous." But, they probably aren't a danger to your health.

Medicine pats itself on the back for the benefits of its cancer regimens. Skin cancer is the most common of all forms, generally easily treated and almost always curable. Its high rate of cure helps with statistics given out regarding the benefit of modern cancer therapy. Skin cancers are easily curable because - except for melanoma which amounts to less than three percent of skin cancers - they are really cancer in name only. But, they keep dermatologists busy and add to their revenue.

Skin cancer is very often a part of the aging process. A common accompaniment. Physicians make a disease out of it. And patients follow suit. It keeps older folks going to the doctor.

Let's go back to the prairie, or most anywhere. You hear hoofbeats approaching, what are you most likely to see coming over the rise?

Horses, of course. Common sense tells you that. You have that common sense. But remember, the medical system has to keep an eye out for zebras. So again, don't forget YOUR common sense when you go to the clinic or hospital. If YOU don't have some, YOU may well miss it when your attending physician is lacking.

Dr. Ed's question might also suggest that WE - you and I - learn how to deal and live with the obvious. "What would that be? What is the obvious?" you ask.

Illness and injury, aches and pains, are part of everyone's life. There is just no getting around it. Name someone who has lived without disease, disability or discomfort. Then, I will tell you that either that person is very young, lived a short life or is good at ignoring problems.

When we hear hoofbeats, we might be prodded to see what's coming towards us in our lives and in our bodies. We CAN learn how to do that. Then, we won't be terribly surprised when our bodies bring us a few more problems and challenges to deal with as we get older.

Common sense simply suggests that when we hear hoofbeats, we prepare for horses. A Shrewd Physician follows that simple notion.

Scientific Medicine

You might think, "This talk about heart and head, common sense and compassion is all well and good. But, isn't medicine a scientific pursuit? First and foremost? Isn't it more scientific, rather than artistic, especially since we live in a time of scientific study and technological advancement?" Good questions.

Early in my medical career I attended an annual convention of the American Holistic Medical Association in La Crosse, Wisconsin. In preparation for that particular meeting, the founding president, Dr. Norman Shealy, sent letters to the deans of all (about 100 at the time) American medical and osteopathic schools.

In his letters, he asked a simple and direction question: "What is scientific medicine?"

Dr. Shealy received a handful of responses, most of which were on the order of: "That's an interesting question. We ought to do some research on it." Really?!

Those who replied to Shealy's question were invited to address the convention on the topic. Five accepted. Yet, not one of them dared to address the subject directly. Instead, they merely concurred that IT was an important issue before going off on tangents to talk of their school's own particular interests and work. They were unwilling or unprepared to confront the issue head on.

But, really? Whether it is declared loudly or not, medicine clearly claims to base its practices on science - practically the whole medical curriculum is one "science" or another - and physicians claim to use the best of science and technology.

The phrase "art of medicine" is rarely heard in medical training, while science, science and more science is pushed into students' brains. The large majority of students have taken a college major in one scientific field or another. Few of the artistically inclined are drawn into the field (an applicant has to take a host of science and math courses just to meet entrance requirements which weeds out many) and there is less and less talk of artistry in the profession as the years pass. Still, the majority of modern medicine is neither scientific nor artistic.

Much scientific research has been done over the past two centuries from which medicine contends to draw and provide rationale for its philosophy and practice. But, a large swath of medical functions are dictated by tradition: "That's the way we have been doing it for years." By consensus: "That's what they taught us in medical school, right or wrong." By the latest drug on the market: "Here are some samples of a hot new medication. Give these a try." By personal preference: "I like this method. It usually works for me." By faith in authority: "We wouldn't steer you wrong. Would we?"

The "science" involved in medicine changes from day to day and year to year as medicine tries to delve more and more deeply into the molecules and genetics of its human subjects. Yet after spending trillions of dollars in research on major diseases over recent decades, little progress has been made toward "cures."

Often, the forest gets lost for the trees. Physicians dwell on "science" and end up treating cells and tissues instead of humans, tests rather than patients.

The focus of treatment shifts and changes with the winds of research. Merely reflect on how one year we are supposed to eat butter and the next margarine. One medication is in vogue for a time and then a newer one is on the market, soon to be replaced by another. The media touts a new regimen for this disease or that. Often, the previous highly-praised medication has been found over time to have adverse effects upon an organ system remote from the intended target.

Sadly, it seems that the science of medicine is akin to the science of warfare. "Go out and hunt the enemy. Destroy it by any method available." In the case of modern medicine, chemicals and knives are the weapons of choice with radiation coming in a distant third. Yet, we know that therapeutic weapons often disturb and destroy normal body cells and functions. We very often trade one problem for another.

In Vietnam, we destroyed villages to save the country. In Medicine, we destroy body defenses (blood cells, specifically) to save the whole body. But, neither approach seems to work very well. Whatever medical science brings forth, it gets displaced with something newer and seemingly more elegant. But often, far removed from the real world of real human beings.

The story is told that many decades ago the Dean of the Harvard Medical School used to meet with and speak to the incoming freshman class on their first day. He gave the same pep talk each year and always threw in the proviso about their medical education, "Fifty percent of what we teach you here will be outdated in the next twenty years. The problem is that we don't know which fifty percent that is."

Well, that problem does persist despite scientific discoveries, technological advancement, and media propaganda. Science is only part of the answer for the needs of society in general and for medicine and the patients it is called to serve.

Science is often necessary in medical practice and care. But, prudent patients and practitioners recognize that the verdict is still out on so many of the ills of mankind. There is still much room for common sense and compassion while medicine is just beginning to understand the depth and wonder of the human being.

Interestingly, a large part of scientific medicine should be considered experimental. And not just with problems like cancer. Since most often your physician really, honestly, and truly doesn't know what is causing your problem, his/her prescribed treatment is on the order of an experiment. That's why your physician is wont to say, "Give this medication a try."

Even when the supposed cause is known, the full effects of the treatment is surely unknown because every patient is different. Sounds like an experiment to me.

We generally imagine medicine to be a science, an art and an ethical profession. One backed by a creed and a philosophy. It is generally thought that physicians upon graduation from medical school take a binding oath to uphold the creed and treat patients in an ethical if not sacred manner. That way of the ancients was made objective through the Oaths of Hippocrates and Maimonides. (See Appendix for originals.)

But by the 1920s, only one quarter of American medical schools administered any kind of oath on graduation. I took no oath nor ever had a single class in the history of medicine. I don't recall ever hearing the name Hippocrates spoken in my studies. He was old, dated and irrelevant by the time I sat in medical school.

Hippocratic Oath (a modern version):

I swear to fulfill, to the best of my ability and judgment, this covenant:

I will respect the hard-won scientific gains of those physicians in whose steps I walk, and gladly share such knowledge as is mine with those who are to follow.

I will apply, for the benefit of the sick, all measures [that] are required, avoiding those twin traps of overtreatment and therapeutic nihilism.

I will remember that there is art to medicine as well as science, and that warmth, sympathy, and understanding may outweigh the surgeon's knife or the chemist's drug.

I will not be ashamed to say "I know not," nor will I fail to call in my colleagues when the skills of another are needed for a patient's recovery.

I will respect the privacy of my patients, for their problems are not disclosed to me that the world may know. Most especially must I tread with care in matters of life and death. If it is given to me to save a life, all thanks. But it may also be within my power to take a life; this awesome responsibility must be faced with great humbleness and awareness of my own frailty. Above all, I must not play at God.

I will remember that I do not treat a fever chart, a cancerous growth, but a sick human being, whose illness may affect the person's family and economic stability. My responsibility includes these related problems, if I am to care adequately for the sick.

I will prevent disease whenever I can, for prevention is preferable to cure.

I will remember that I remain a member of society, with special obligations to all my fellow human beings, those sound of mind and body as well as the infirm.

If I do not violate this oath, may I enjoy life and art, respected while I live and remembered with affection thereafter. May I always act so as to preserve the finest traditions of my calling and may I long experience the joy of healing those who seek my help.

This modern version of the Hippocratic Oath, penned by Dr. Louis Lasagna, had not found a place in Texas medical education as of my graduation in 1977. Yet, it seems there has been a push in recent years to pay some homage to the ancient vow - at least at the moment of graduation. According to one survey done in 1993, 98 percent of American medical and osteopathic schools were then administering an oath of some kind, the majority based on the words of Hippocrates. But, I wonder how many students are forewarned and do so thoughtfully or just to get their sheepskin.

As the oath is presently stated above, it is hard to see anyone objecting. And any physician who was guided thus would do so quite honorably by Hippocrates. S/he would likely have real potential for becoming a Frugal Physician as well.

Medicine does have traditions, but most of them date back to recent generations and the scientific era. The ancients - their history and beliefs - generally hold little importance as do other seemingly significant influences on human lives, such as business and finances, nutrition and exercise, religion and spirit.

Oaths taken past and present are laudable. But, I suspect modern medical education still does not stack up to those idealistic words of Hippocrates and modern imitators. 21st century medical curricula are little changed from a generation past. Placing huge emphasis on the body, "scientific" disciplines, and disease (pathology), medical education continues to give short shrift to mind and spirit, health and healing, and many real life common sense issues.

Science and technology surely hold sway in medicine and will continue so as long as we humans continue our materialistic ways. The big "University Hospital" is its most notable symbol. That being the case tells reams about the state of modern medicine.

University Medicine cares for the worst of the worst with the best, fastest and most expensive technology. These centers which provide tertiary care are last down the road from front line clinics and small hospitals. Such places have trauma centers, intensive care units, facilities for high risk infants and the like. But, they are hardly like being "down home."

New physicians come out of such institutions prepared for and imagining the worst scenarios, and often helping to create them. The vast majority of time, they meet the mundane which they have not been prepared for. Your physician, if s/he is like most, really has not been prepared for real people and real life medicine. That is another very simple reason that medicine is out of hand, physicians magnify and exaggerate, and disease care is very expensive.

A typical western medical curriculum is outlined below. This program is exactly the same as it was more than a generation ago.

First Year: Anatomy, Biochemistry, Cell Biology, Embryology, Genetics, Human Behavior, Immunology, Neuroscience, General Physiology

Second Year: Microbiology, Pathology, Pharmacology, Clinical Medicine, Pre-Clinical Electives

Third Year: Family Medicine, Internal Medicine, Obstetrics and Gynecology, Pediatrics, Psychiatry, Surgery

Fourth Year: Acute Care, Ambulatory Care, Electives, Medicine Subinternship

There are huge gaps in medical education as you might guess by studying the curriculum above. Science and technology, cells and organs, body and disease hold court to the exclusion or near exclusion of so many other aspects of human life.

You might think an education is meant to put the graduate on his/her feet with knowledge and experience to proceed in learning and discovery in the coming days. The fresh graduate has learned a lot of names and diseases and diagnoses and drugs. But since human life and death, health and pain, and many other things come into the hands of a new physician, it seems that some of those gaps might deserve being addressed.

I am reminded of my first graduation - from high school - eleven years before the medical event. Actually, it was graduation rehearsal and we were being led through the planned program. Dr. Senne, our principal, took great pains to let us know, "We have prepared a perfect graduation ceremony for you. Please cooperate and do your part."

I could not help but think aloud and mutter into the ear of my neighbor, "I would much rather he had worked on a perfect education."

Hippocrates pointed students and physicians in the right direction. Patients and the public can learn quite a bit by just reading and pondering the Hippocratic Oath and looking to see how well their health care providers subscribe to it. Sadly, too many of Dr. Hippocrates's common sense suggestions and injunctions have gotten lost or crowded out along the way.

Our society and our medical care providers must strive to better understand relatively simple and obvious concepts of life and health, regardless of their being scientific or not. Else, orthodox medicine will continue on its expensive, materialistic, and very wasteful ways.

A Frugal Physician uses science when called for. S/he realizes, however, that the human organism is a miniature of the whole - body, mind and spirit. This fact makes for a large vista - far more expansive than modern science - to be surveyed when dealing with many if not all human ills.

Routine Tests

The most valuable thing I ever heard spoken when I was in medical school came from the lips of Dr. Cheves Smythe, who was the first Dean of our medical school. Dr. Smythe was an internist and geriatrician and later (after I graduated) Chief of Medicine for the school. He made rounds with us one day when I was on the Internal Medicine Service at St. Joseph's Hospital.

This was the only time I ever saw or heard Dr. Smythe in action: one of the few high points of my medical school career. I was very impressed and wished he had made rounds regularly. Smythe seemed to be a medical wiz, down to earth and artful. He made two comments in the midst of our informal session that I most certainly will never forget.

In the midst of his brief lesson, the slim Boston-accented and bow-tied Smythe said, "Ninety percent of useful information should come from the physical examination and history you do on your patients." Well, I agreed. But even in the 1970s, medical testing certainly seemed to take up a lot more than 10 percent of our time and the patients' money.

I later learned that that practice was hardly new, dating from the 1940s. That was when Tinsley Harrison, the famed editor of *Harrison's Textbook of Internal Medicine*, made a crisp comment worthy of attention in any decade. Harrison was disturbed even then about "the present-day tendency towards a five-minute history followed by a five-day barrage of special tests in the hope that the diagnostic rabbit may suddenly emerge from the laboratory hat."

Dr. Smythe seemed to follow Tinsley's lead as he went on to announce that, "You should only order a lab test or Xray when you know what the result will be. And then, if you know what the result will be, you quite probably don't have to order the test."

He was saying that a physician should have a good idea of what s/he is looking for when ordering tests. Instead, batteries of tests are often done willy nilly with little thought of results or costs. Such was and is likely still the norm.

One of my earliest real life medical school memories comes from my first year. Long before I encountered Dr. Smythe, I met Dr. Sperling. There was a huge difference between the two. I was assigned to spend one afternoon a week in Sperling's family practice clinic on the north side of Houston. Every student was given the opportunity to get his/her feet wet and also get out of the classroom while looking over the shoulder of a primary care physician during that first year.

Fortunately or not, I was assigned to Dr. Gerald Sperling. I probably prejudiced myself against him early on. The physician was a literally bulging, red-haired man in his 40s. He was very large - around 300 pounds - even though he had recently had stomach stapling surgery and lost much weight, I was told by one of his staff. That didn't sit comfortably within me, as I have long thought that physicians and other medical professionals should at least try to set examples for their patients and clients. Well, that made it tough for Dr. Sperling to impress me positively. He had one strike against him immediately.

Quickly, I noticed a pattern in the doctor's work. He seemed to prescribe gamma globulin quite liberally. You name the problem, a gamma globulin shot would help. He was ordering lots of lab tests. Both surely increased his income. Strike 2.

One particular consult was with a young man with some general complaints. The doctor did the usual "brief history and cursory examination" and ordered a number of tests. Some moments later, the nurse came into the doctor's office where I sat in a corner biding my time.

She remarked, "The new patient is concerned about the costs of the tests you have ordered for him. He is paying out of pocket and has limited funds."

Doctor Sperling moved away from the Wall Street Journal on his desk. He walked over with the nurse towards the door and whispered to her, "Just negotiate with him." Strike 3.

That was enough for me. It seemed clear that Sperling was more a businessman than a medical professional. It wasn't long before I made an appointment to speak with the dean of the medical school and told him of my experiences at Dr. Sperling's office, my impressions and discomfort with his practice. He listened carefully and sent me on.

Before long, I received a note from the Office of the Dean telling me, "You need not continue your Primary Care Practicum. You will be given credit, however, for completing it."

It was not the school's "business" to tell Dr. Sperling how to practice. UTMSH may or may not have sent him any more preceptees, but it certainly would not have bothered him about "negotiating" on blood tests.

A Frugal Physician recognizes reasons to limit testing and prescribing, but modern medicine pretty much holds to the axiom: "It is always better to do too many tests, than not enough. And it is certainly better to prescribe too many drugs, than too few."

In *Confessions of A Medical Heretic*, Dr. Robert Mendelsohn relates "... one of my key pieces of subversive advice to medical students is this: To pass an exam, get through medical school, and retain your sanity, always choose the most interventionist answer." That was not his way. But, he knew the ways of medicine and that ordering tests, doing procedures, and prescribing would rarely be faulted in the modern era.

In my own career, I followed Dr. Smythe's advice. I used tests quite sparingly. When I ran a troop medical clinic at Fort Riley, Kansas, I overheard more than a few times, "The doc hardly ever orders a lab test." The technicians and physician assistants thought it quite unusual.

I figured it wasn't my job to keep the lab techs at the hospital busy. I'm sure they already had plenty of work to do.

The age group with which I worked, mostly young soldiers - 20 to 40, and mostly in the lower end of that range, were very unlikely to have anything seriously abnormal show up on any medical test.

A Wise Physician knows the limitations of tests, that they are hugely overdone, and that most patient populations can get along quite nicely with a tenth of the procedures that are now done. Therefore, they should be ordered much less frequently. Only when indications are clear. They still may be unnecessary (remember Dr. Smythe) because the results may well be predictable or because those results may not affect any potential treatment plan.

There are, however, other reasons to do medical tests beyond getting information in search of a diagnosis. One such reason brings a story to mind from the experience of this once young physician. It may be instructive from a number of angles.

I dropped the ball a few obvious times in my career. One occasion sticks in my memory when a young enlisted man came to the clinic complaining of chest discomfort. He was obviously in more than physical distress. It didn't take long for me to find out that his favorite uncle had just died after a heart attack.

The young man was scared and wanted his heart tested. I tried on two or three visits to reassure him that, "You're too young to have a heart attack. You're on duty, working, and in obviously good health. Your exam is perfectly normal. You have had a shock because of your uncle's death. You need to grieve a bit and just let things settle. You will be fine."

Well, things weren't going to be fine because this physician didn't listen to his patient. The young man persisted making trips to the clinic until a day came when I was off duty. The practitioner who was ON DUTY - and paying attention - that day decided, "The only way to appease this fellow is do what he asks. Let's get a therapeutic EKG."

The EKG was surely WNL - Within Normal Limits. The soldier was satisfied. Maybe cured. And we heard nothing more from him.

Listening to the patient can be even more valuable than talking with him/her. And sometimes, just the administration of a test can be therapeutic. A lesson worth learning.

Normal?

Within Normal Limits, WNL, Normal Range, or just simply Normal. Most laboratory test results come back in numbers, but physicians almost always consider them with respect to "Normal."

But, what is Normal? A friend used to tell me that, "Normal is a setting on a dryer." Cute. But, at least worth a moment's pause.

If a doctor orders tests, s/he has to have some idea what normal is.

Doesn't s/he?

We have already addressed the idea that s/he probably doesn't have to order as many tests as the next physician. Certainly, a Prudent Physician doesn't while the rest order ten times as many.

Nonetheless in the modern world, your physician is likely to recommend tests sooner or later, more or less. That was what s/he was taught to do. Dr. Smythe wasn't teaching regularly and in all med schools around the country. I'm sure most of my fellow students didn't pay much attention to what he said, anyway. He was pretty much alone in that approach to medicine.

Medical tests are in vogue. They are almost as important as the concept of disease itself. In fact, physicians seem to thrive on tests. If you look through most patient charts, past and present, you will see that much of their bulk comes from test forms and results.

The weights and proportions of documents in a patient's chart offer clear hints. They tell about the physician's interests and what s/he values in different aspects of his/her work.

This reminds me of the old idea of surveying a town to tell what the people living there value most. Think about that for moment, if you will. In past times, what were the largest buildings constructed? Then, think again about modern cities. Which buildings rise up above the rest?

It used to be that churches and schools were most prominent. Now in most cities, you will see that banks, government buildings, insurance companies, investment offices, and hospitals have outgrown their neighbors.

In a similar way, test forms and results have overgrown patient charts. History and physical exam and commentary about the patient most generally take second place in time and value.

Doctors lean on tests for a number of reasons, like:

• They are taught about them from the beginning of medical school. Testing gets about as much credence as pathology and diagnosis in training. They see residents and staff people ordering and ordering on the wards and in clinics in the latter years of medical school.

- Lab tests almost always have objective results, suggesting right or wrong, good or bad, normal or abnormal. Numbers on paper are almost "tangible" and are supportive in medical detective work. Much more so than hunches, intuitions, and subjective observations. Physicians are scientifically and mathematically minded. They are problem solvers, or endeavor to be. Like Sherlock Holmes, medical investigators need objective clues toward making diagnoses. Intuition has little to do with most medical practice.

Many practitioners will tell you medicine is meant to be an objective process. I have to admit that, in college, I turned from a double major including English to studying Medical Technology alone. In part because my first English professor gave me a B and said, "You write like a radio commentator."

He was probably right. Regardless, I decided, "I don't need his subjective grading. I am going to focus on science, get a degree in an area where the questions and answers are clear cut. I don't like these subjective critiques. What does he know, anyway?"

Well, I have learned otherwise over the course of the years. Medicine, like life, is rarely cut-and-dried, black and white. But rather shaded in grays or mixtures of colors.

Of the dozens of courses we took in medical school, only two gave essay bordering on subjective tests. Interestingly to my way of thinking, they were the best courses in the whole curriculum. The Biochemistry and Reproductive Biology Departments had teaching programs and general principles of operation which promoted thinking. Imagine that! Thinking was supported in at least some courses of study in the medical curriculum.

- Physicians like to use quantitative tests because they help to PROVE things. Proof is important in medicine and in science.

Unfortunately, it is very difficult to prove most things even with objective, numerical tests. Robert Mendelsohn tells of his favorite study "in which 197 of 200 (patients) were 'cured' of their abnormalities simply by repeating their lab tests!"

There are so many variables involved in blood testing and similar procedures, some physicians ignore or don't even consider:

1) Testing technology is not flawless. Equipment makes errors. This is less common than in past years but still happens.

2) Humans make mistakes in preparing specimens. This is not uncommon. John Doe's sample gets mixed up with Mary Smith's. It's certainly more common than babies getting placed with the wrong mothers, which is hard for most of us to imagine. Yet true and still happens. Mistakes and mishaps occur everywhere.

3) Test results vary from day to day and hour to hour, and depend on many factors. That is one reason you are supposed to be fasting before submitting to a number of blood tests. Blood pressure monitoring is particularly apt to be "labile" because of place and time and the person taking the reading. If you want your blood pressure to go down, leave the doctor's office.

4) Just taking a test, probing the body with a needle or an electronic device can influence human chemistry and reactions enough to alter test results. Especially in more sensitive patients.

5) Patients are also influenced for good or ill by the technicians doing the tests. This is called Observer Effect. Expectations of patient and physician do affect outcomes in clinic and hospital.

6) Physicians commonly "throw out" test results that don't fit with their often preconceived views of "what is really wrong with the patient." How many of the test reports pasted or printed into your chart have your physician either forgotten to read, ignored, or decided, "Well, that can't be right. It doesn't fit the pattern at all."

7) Many test reports are never even read. They just get filed.

• Working with theoretically straightforward tests and their results is a whole lot easier than relating to patients with their varied needs, concerns, and idiosyncrasies. Real Physicians develop sensitivity and understanding of human psychology. But, psychology and counsel are low on many physicians' medical totem pole because practice focuses so heavily on body physiology.

Is a test the key to sorting out a patient's life and illness? A test certainly may bring real information, but human beings are more than collections of body parts and results of tests meant to evaluate their function.

A Real Physician gets to know patients as human beings first. That takes many qualities that are not taught or broached in medical school. Medical training is still an objective, numbers-oriented, quantitative process. But, a Frugal Physician uses tests carefully and only to back up his/her less than perfect ability and execution.

NORMAL may not be important in your case. Unless you are a setting on a dryer. You may be Supernormal or Abnormal or Off the Scale to begin with. So, does it really matter whether your test results are Within Normal Limits, or not? Tests don't define people, unless we let them.

A Frugal Physician strives to get a sense of your very nature, not just your biological form. If a test has something to do with that larger nature, well and good.

Xray, Xray! Read All About It!

Most people in any business or profession are average in their work. If you want an Average Physician, you have many to choose from. You get just Average Care. The care may be technically correct, but then your practitioner is more a technician than a physician. Think about it.

Most physicians, being technicians, are practiced at ordering and reviewing tests (mostly blood and urine). They also request Xrays which are usually "read" by specialists called radiologists (Xray Doctors). Physicians get reports from radiologists and all they have to do is "read" what has been dictated onto the report form.

Interestingly, a number of studies have been done over the years showing that there can be wide discrepancies in interpretation of Xrays. Xray reading is not as cut and dried as blood testing in which machines do all the calculation. Reports can change in up to 20 percent of cases when Xrays are re-read by the SAME radiologist. There is clearly a large subjective element dependent on the "eye of the beholder." In this case, the Xray Physician. S/he "reads your Xrays." The "reading" of any physical test or scan is subject to interpretation and error.

Mendelsohn, the Medical Heretic, called the Xray machine "the most pervasive and most dangerous tool in the doctor's office." Now three decades later, Xray machines are not quite as common in small medical offices. They have gotten more sophisticated and expensive. But, the fact that many physicians don't have them on their premises doesn't make them any less worrisome.

Xrays and the related radioactivity of elements were discovered at the end of the 19th century. Those events created great stirs in the scientific world and spawned the development of many tools for use in medical practice. Some continue to this day, while many others have disappeared except in museums and texts on the advancement of medical technology.

In recent times, Xrays have spawned many imaging systems - too many to mention - including CT Scans and MRI Scans. The former is a computerized version of Xray and the latter uses magnets and radio frequency fields to produce pictures of internal organs. They are "bigger and better" and bring much higher charges with their now very common use. Expensive equipment (starting at over a million dollars) requires commensurate pricing.

Guess who pays? You pay well. Simple studies begin around $500 and can run up to ten times that amount. CT Scans are usually less costly, but no bargain.

Even from the orthodox view, Xrays and medical radiation have not always been beneficial. Numerous ill effects as well as secondary disease and death have resulted from their use. That is all supposedly now in the past. How can we really know?

Over a hundred years since their introduction, Xrays and scanning devices still create an aura of power for Radiologic and Regular Physicians with radiographs (Xrays) in hand. "Magic in medicine. Wow! They can see inside my body. That tells them what's really going on. Amazing."

So, they might wish. And so they might like you to think.

• You might wonder what an Xray really shows. "Does it really photograph the inside of my body? Can physicians see things as they really are with Xrays?"

Yes and No. Mostly, No. There is no device known to man that can see inside a body exactly as it exists, moves and breathes. Xrays and similar devices create shadows and contrasts which make bones and organs stand out against the other tissues nearby. Computers enhance images and make them more "readable."

Still, those shadows can be deceptive as much as revealing. That's where interpretation comes in and also where error or over-reading can happen.

Furthermore, Xrays are physical tests which only picture one dimension of the human form. Others lie yet hidden from the eyes of the Regular Physician however magical his testing and devices may appear.

• Xrays pick up where blood tests leave off. They are used by all kinds of physicians and dentists, podiatrists and chiropractors. But, Xrays characterize the surgeon as blood work does the internist. Between the two tools, physicians expect to diagnose most ailments. But, it often doesn't work out quite that way.

Most human ailments don't show up on an Xray, blood test, EKG, culture, or scan. Only a tiny portion do. Probably less the one percent. Nonetheless, since physicians are body oriented, they will continue to look and look for the source of illness in physical tests. Until found, they run the gamut. Failing to find what they are looking for in the body, they may well figure that the problem has to be psychological.

I remember listening to a patient marveling about how detailed and determined her doctor was: "Oh, my land. He leaves no stone unturned. He has ordered everything he can think of. Doctor hasn't got my condition figured out quite yet. But, not for lack of trying. He is so thorough." Don't you wonder about the size of the bill!?

• Xrays and tests are prolific. They breed and breed again. One procedure leads to another.

This is in a general as well as specific sense. As medicine specializes, it tends to complicate things. More specialties, more diseases, more potential diagnoses, more tests. And then tests within tests. "Fractionate those enzymes." "Subculture those bacteria." "Get some more films (Xrays) of that extremity."

On a single patient basis, one chest Xray leads to another. I remember how heavy old Xray films used to be. Lugging the Xray folders of some patients used to be akin to a weight lifting exercise.

The last time I went to the dentist, 18 different Xrays were done on my little mouth. I only had 30 teeth at the time, four of which were in a bridge and another under a crown. "More than a little overkill," I thought. But, I watched it go by.

I felt outside my element in the dentist chair, especially since I hadn't sat there for several years. I learned a lesson that dentists are in more ways than I had imagined: Regular Physicians in Disguise. Maybe someone with dental experience will write a followup to this effort *In Search of A Frugal Dentist*.

- No Xray or test is totally innocuous. That is why your Xray Physician and Technicians always wear leaded aprons to protect themselves while they "shoot you."

They figure that the benefits of doing the Xray outweigh the risks. The risks may be minimal, but we might wonder more about the potential benefits.

Radiologists don't order Xrays. They do radiological exams on request of other physicians. They rarely question those orders since they make money thanks to other physicians who decide "we need those films."

- Computerized Xrays and Scans have gotten very expensive. "Well, the equipment really is expensive. And, we have to pay for technician and radiologist time, you know."

I have often reflected about the development of these new technologies. They were just appearing when I was finishing medical training in the late 70s. Plain old Xrays were common, EKGs, EEGs, ultrasound and a few other simple scans. Now, there is a plethora of choices with technicians for each device and high prices to go along.

A medical friend who works in a small hospital told me recently of being button-holed by the hospital administrator who had a patient chart in hand. The administrator asked my friend, "Why didn't you order a CT scan on this patient?" Rather than address the question directly, the medic merely responded, "What medical school did you attend?" The administrator quickly changed the conversation, but the implication was clear. More money was needed in the medical coffers. But, my friend was trying to serve his patient rather than promote business.

The obvious overall question arises with regard to the larger gamut of medical technology: Have these new and expensive devices, and their growing use, shown forth benefits at any level commensurate to the cost of their development and even the cost of their routine use? Let's put it another way: Has the patient public become healthier or less diseased since the medical profession has latched onto these very expensive and very commonly used devices? You might wonder.

• In the midst of writing this book, I had a significant injury which taught me a few things. I fell from a ladder, my right foot landing in a hole and my ankle ballooning such that I was laid up for weeks. I remember remarking to friends on two different occasions in the days before the incident; "I have worked from ladders for years and never fallen." I watched the words come out of my mouth. I know better than to say NEVER.

The injury was serious and painful. The ankle was bloated so that I could barely get around with a cane. I spent weeks on the couch.

One friend told me about his recent ankle injury. An ER visit, an Xray and plastic boot for his ankle cost him $1600. And that was just the beginning.

My neighbor watched me hobbling around from across the fence and repeatedly asked, "Do you think it's broken? I bet you it's broken." He and others kept hinting, suggesting, telling me that I needed an Xray.

My response was "We'll never know." What would a Xray tell me that I needed to know. Had a bone protruded from the skin after the fall, I would have sought emergency attention.
But with the structure outwardly intact,

- I had firm trust that Nature would handle the problem quite well. Fractured, sprained, or otherwise. It would just take time. And, it did. Six weeks to get around without a cane. Three months to feel at ease walking. Six months before I sometimes felt the injured foot was doing better than the other.
- I figured Xrays and a medical visit would give limited information and just cost money which I did not have to spend. Still, the information may have been sufficient to make a physician want to intervene in one way or another and expend more money.
- I knew that the foot is not just bone, but ligaments, tendons, fascia, vessels, nerves, lymphatics, sheaths, skin, and other layers totally invisible to Xrays or knives or the searching eyes behind them.
- I understood that my bodily forces knew much better how to put things back in order than any physician, with or without Xrays. They created that foot decades ago following some arcane pattern. They certainly could do it again.
- I was confident that "Nature heals and the doctor takes the fee." I took the time to let Nature do her work. The doctor was deemed unnecessary because the patient was aware of some of the layers of the healing process.

A Frugal Physician recognizes that there is no magic in Xrays, even though they have a mystique. They are just another test. Their use should be thought out carefully before an order is given. And if the results are anticipated ahead of time (Dr. Smythe again), they often may be dispensed with.

Having looked at Xrays from some critical angles, I have to admit that there are novel uses of Xrays. I learned about them in my internship. Curiously, these were totally unexpected results of otherwise routine Xrays. Two such come to mind.

The first concerns Dr. Gus Wood, a fellow Family Practice resident, whom you will read more about in the Teaching and Learning chapter. As I recall it, Gus had an accident of some sort. "Banged his head" and became a little disoriented. He got himself attended to and the Attending Physician decided he should have Xrays. A Skull Series was ordered even though by the time Gus was seen he was back in working order.

The test results took a few days to come back because the radiologist was off for the weekend. It appears that the radiologist had some outside help when he read Gus's films. After the report was dictated and typed up, it was freely circulated among the residents. It read something to this effect: "The cranial vault and associated structures show no significant abnormalities. There is however an opacity consistent with a fecalith in the Circle of Willis which has likely been present for many years and may not be considered abnormal for this subject." I will let the reader conjure the implications of a "fecalith in the Circle of Willis."

The second incident had some similarities and involved myself. I had finished the first year of Family Practice Residency and decided that was enough for me. Subsequently, I was assigned to undergo a six-week Flight Surgeon training in Fort Rucker, Alabama. You guessed it. I had to have a Flight Physical which included a standard chest Xray.

That Xray report came back with better results than Gus's. The radiologist pronounced: "AP and Lateral views of the chest reveal no abnormalities of heart, lungs or rib cage. There are, however, clear suggestions of vestigial wing buds. This man is ready to fly."

Rocket Science

We bow to technology in the modern era, like we did to religion and the divine right of kings in ages past. In the medical arena, this has been somewhat aptly called Faith in Saint Johns Hopkins, referring to the highly revered hospital and medical school in Baltimore. (See Anything

Can Cure Anything.)

Saint Johns Hopkins achieved its reputation decades before scientific technology exploded. Awe inspired in such institutions has grown and grown over the years. I remember walking across the Texas Medical Center in Houston some months before I entered medical school. The TMC Campus was huge. Looming like a big city, covering blocks and blocks, and rising higher and higher with new hospitals and additions thereto. I have not returned since graduating in 1977, but I am sure Texas Medical Center has substantially expanded horizontally and vertically, mystically and financially for the ever faithful since those days.

Similar changes have occurred in other large and not so large cities across the western world. Whole corridors and sections of towns have uprooted residential areas to create wall-to-wall medical facilities and ancillary structures, parking lots and garages.

The nearest medical complex to the author in Billings, Montana (pop. 100,000), has recently erected its second Cancer Center. This is surely a tribute to medical technology, but not necessarily medical progress. The center is devoted to treatment of cancer. If decades-long and deep-pocket medical efforts to deal with that dread disease had been at all successful, one would think that smaller and fewer facilities would be in order. But, time marches on and Almighty Technology continues to expand, if not advance.

I am reminded of a number of visits which Dr. Charles Berry made to speak at our medical school. Berry had been Director of Medical Operations and Research at the Manned Spacecraft Center (Houston, Texas) during the Gemini and Apollo programs. He also had many other titles including professor of our medical school.

Berry had been deeply involved in medical preparations for early space voyages. He talked about risks of space flight as well as opportunities and benefits which America had accrued from manned space ventures. He also made attempts to suggest that the future of human medicine was bound to have successes similar to those of space medicine. Essentially, he was saying, "If we can conquer outer space, we can overcome illness."

But, I have to say that human medicine and rocket science stand far apart. We used to say, "Medicine is not rocket science." Students don't need to be geniuses to get through training and pass off as Regular Physicians. Nor do most medical processes require the precision of a shuttle launch.

Still, I think sometimes that even "Rocket science isn't rocket science." The space program has months, years, and decades to prepare for anticipated needs and possible problems in launch, orbit, and reentry. Systems are redundant upon redundant. But, rockets and shuttles are likely never as complicated as human beings. Simply because they are machines and not living beings.

We certainly have had space successes. However, Dr. Berry spoke to us long before the Challenger and Columbia Space Shuttle disasters. There are times and seasons for success and failure in space exploration and in medical ventures. Technology has been in season for many decades now. While its time is not over, its potency is surely beginning to wane. New forces will and must take charge and bring balance to practically all disciplines in the modern world. Thinking back to the Texas Medical Center and Johnson Manned Spacecraft Center causes me to be reminded of another phenomenon of particular interest in the 70s and 80s. That is the acclaimed and sometimes worshipped television and later film series called *Star Trek*.

The Starship Enterprise cruised the known universe and took on all comers, like the Lone Ranger did in an earlier era. Instead of using a horse and six-shooter, the Enterprise had 23rd century technology so the crew could travel at time warp speed, go into battle with laser weapons, and translocate personnel on rays of light. I have to admit that I was never a Star Trek fan. I did see one or two Star Trek films and seriously put it to the test of my critical eye. The reader should also know that friends used to have a difficult time when we went to movies together, especially when there were medical parts to the film. I couldn't help myself. I would grumble out louder than a whisper, "Ah, it would never happen like that. Didn't they have a medical consultant for this movie?" I would get nudged and asked to pipe down.

One of my especial upsets has been about movie blood. Many films botch bloody scenes. Why can't they make fake blood look like real blood rather than thin paint or thick Koolaid?

In the one Star Trek film I recall, *The Undiscovered Country*, a violent scene occurred involving the Klingons. Gorkon, one of their potentates, was spurting blood and dying in front of the Klingon crew. The Klingons, though they looked quite human, had purple blood among other differences with the Enterprise crew. But, blood color wasn't the main problem.

The leader of the Klingons was bleeding to death. After a few ineffectual preliminaries with scanning devices, aging Dr. Bones McCoy jumped in and started beating on the bleeding Gorkon's chest to revive the Klingon.

First things first. Stop the bleeding. Everybody knows that. Even grade schoolers. No amount of resuscitation efforts will overcome loss of blood. Even Klingon blood!

But, there was another obvious and critical point. At least, it was to me, and fits our theme. The Starship was spanning the galaxies three hundred years hence using the latest technologies, but space medicine was still using 20th century first aid. How lame! If they could respond to "Beam me up, Scottie," the Enterprise crew certainly should have passed beyond the stage of mouth-to-mouth resuscitation and closed cardiac massage.

Three hundred years from now, we ought to do better than that. But, maybe not. Consider how well we are doing now with all of our 21st century technology.

Where are the medical marvels? Oh, there are a few. Very few. But, most of them don't filter down to make much difference in the daily lives of the great majority of patients.

Part of the problem is simply that science and physicians still don't understand human beings. "Human beings are not machines. Nor do they respond like machines." Technologists act as if everything can be approached in "machine mode."

Certainly, we have machine-like qualities and can do many things better than any robot. But, we also emulate chemical factories. The human form makes and processes thousands, maybe millions of chemicals. Probably more than all the manufacturing plants in the whole world have ever produced.

The human frame is a veritable "garden of eden" of flora and fauna. Although they are invisible to the naked eye, trillions of microscopic plants and animals - bacteria, viruses, fungi, etc. - live on the surface and within the human body.

That form is also like a miniature magical physics laboratory. It has fantastic electrical networks. The brain itself has more connections than all the world's telephone systems and is capable of using millions of interconnections in any moment.

All aspects of nature can be found within the human being. Much more than science has been able to uncover with present means. We have yet "to boldly go where no man has gone before." The human race really won't create true science and technology until we understand the wonder of the human form. "If not here, then nowhere. If here, then everywhere." Know thy self.

Clinic Visits

In the meantime, we are constrained to the present medical paradigm which does have its good points. Along with the not so good and decidedly bad ones.

The bulk of medicine is practiced in offices and clinics. While those venues are more modern and up-to-date than in generations past, I suspect most of them still exhibit typical shortcomings.

Hospitals have to keep up with inspectors from many angles. Medical offices don't. Interesting isn't it that so many businesses and institutions in the present era are subject to inspection and evaluation from all sorts of directions, but your physician has probably never had his/her office and practice examined. Unless someone has registered a complaint.

The average patient probably wouldn't notice any problems. General appearance and cleanliness likely would be acceptable to most any eye.

But, there are obvious shortfalls in most clinics. Behind the seemingly staid, neat, and orderly facade, many things might be worth the consumer-patient being made aware.

Some of the following queries may have passed through your mind at one time or another:

- Doesn't this office appointment create an unnatural situation? Something is just not quite right. From the moment you enter the doctor's office - even before. Because "YOU go to the doctor." Yes, house calls are almost extinct, but should that be the case?

An abnormal arrangement has occurred from the very outset. This is not really Within Normal Limits, but we let it pass. Everything regarding your illness is out of context when YOU enter a medical clinic. YOU, the patient, didn't get sick in the doctor's office - although that surely has happened many times. It is not that healthy of a place to spend time. There is no way YOU could even imagine carrying the story of your whole illness with you to the clinic. Even if you tried.

YOU developed your illness not just because of the body which transports you around, but also because of your family and social life, your work and worries, your going out and coming in. Your activity and inactivity. Your spiritual life or lack thereof. Your sex life or lack thereof. Your bank account, empty or bulging.

Only a small portion of your life, the patient's life is at all visible and much of the rest is not very accessible, when YOU pick up and go to the medical clinic.

When YOU take yourself to your doctor's office, YOU unknowingly put both of you at a huge disadvantage in trying to get a handle on your health situation. I know YOU didn't have much of a choice. "Doctor doesn't do house calls. Nobody does house calls." Not totally true, but pretty close.

I am reminded of years ago consulting with a patient. The first thing out of her mouth was, "I'm really sorry, doctor. I missed my last appointment because I was sick." I was the one who should have been sorry. My mates and I should have provided for house calls. (See House Calls.)

- Is your physician really qualified? "Well, s/he must be. The Medical Board wouldn't allow him/her to put up a shingle."

Of course, you're quite right. But, I am asking a deeper question as to whether s/he has the qualifications of aptitude, interest, concern, compassion, willingness to meet you as a human being with problems and pain, anxiety and downright fear. And relate to you in a truly humanistic way.

Did your physician pick up those qualities along the way through medical school and advanced training? Or, is s/he just a trained professional, a medical technician, a regular physician?

If your physician met you at your home, in the park, in the sandwich shoppe, would s/he relate to you as a human being and not just a patient? Can you imagine having such an appointment? Could your doctor? If one could be arranged, you certainly would save money and s/he would get a break from the regular routine.

Is your physician really helping people? Or paying the bills? Or vicariously working out his/her own problems through yours?

- Does your physician suit you? Are the two of you really compatible? Can you "work" together? Or did you make an appointment because s/he was close by or convenient?

I am reminded of my early civilian practice days. I heard more than once secondhand that I didn't quite fit the bill. "He is awfully young. An older physician would have been nice." "I wish he had been a she." "I liked the curly hair, but not the beard."

Those may be superficial things. But if the patient can't get past them, both have a problem. And what if the physician doesn't like his/her patient? That might be even worse.

- What kind of personnel work in the doctor's office? Have they got any qualifications at all? What kind of qualifications should there be for one person to tend to another? Oftentimes, like the secretary in a business office, the most valuable people are those at the front desk. Service starts the moment one enters the office. Often before, through telephone contacts.

How were the medical personnel selected? Did they get hired because they have talent beyond completing some brief training program or exercise or less? Or were they hired because they work for $10 an hour? What prompted them to work in medical care? Are they any healthier than the patients who walk in the door?

- Who are all those people sitting and waiting in the lobby? Aren't they all sick? They look sick. What are YOU doing in a place with all these sick people? Some of the help don't look so good either. If a person doesn't feel sick before s/he goes into a clinic, there is a good chance that s/he will before leaving.

- The exam room is small, two people barely fit. Three is a crowd. With the prices patients pay for services, they should be able to get a comfortable seat in which to consult the expensive physician. The patient usually gets to sit on a exam table. And often, in a gown - barely clothed - even before being greeted by the attending doctor.

I have only twice been in medical offices where patients were not first seen in treatment rooms. One was my own and another was that of a homeopath. Homeopaths are pretty much cerebral. They ask a lot of questions. I don't remember the homeopathic physician doing any kind of examination.

The physician-patient interaction is done largely at the doctor's convenience. Offices are not made for patient comfort. The whole process can be quite demeaning and disturbing. Again, a person presenting to a medical office has a good chance of leaving in worse shape - physically, emotionally and financially.

I have remarked a few times to friends about the POWER of a physician: "How many people can you meet and within ten minutes you will be willing to get naked at their request? And pay to do it?"

Two answers come to mind at the present. I won't try to make a connection. One is a physician, the other is a prostitute.

- Medical appointments are generally very brief. A few minutes with the physician. Much time waiting and more time involved in paperwork, vital signs and testing of one kind or another.

The main concern is the "few minutes" which your doctor gets or takes to come up with a plan. It probably took you more time to get out of bed in the morning than it takes most physicians to hear your story (maybe auscultate and palpate) and come up with a plan of action for your problem.

Patients get used to that way of "doing business." They have expectations that their condition will be addressed quickly and correctly. But, should that be based on the VERY modest time investment made in their life by their physician?

This modus operandi is akin to an auto mechanic who listens to a "noise under the hood" for ten minutes and then does the works. Still, you say, "It seems okay. It's always been this way. I feel like it helps. Something happened. The problem at least hasn't gotten worse. The doctor is a nice fella. He tries. He's got a busy life and lots of things to keep up with. A few minutes with him is enough. I wish I could bake him a cake, fatten him up a bit."

The process works. Or so it seems. Some of the time. If it doesn't, you will be back and give the doctor another crack at your problem. And pay another bill. Less in your pocket and more in your physician's.

- The appointment is short and so is the History and Physical Exam. In medical parlance, it is commonly given as "a *brief* history and a *cursory* physical exam."

The physician has numerous reasons for the brevity of the medical history and exam:

1) "I have a busy day ahead. I have to keep on schedule."
2) "Small problems require only a quick history and exam, maybe not even an exam."
3) "This patient's problem is much the same as the one just left."
4) "This episode is just like the last one."
5) "An exam won't show anything, anyway."
6) "This is just a routine office call."
7) "I'm going to order tests which will tell the tale, regardless."

But, tests don't tell the tale. The patient has almost all of the tale to tell and his/her body-being are the source of the tale. Dr. Smythe (see Routine Tests) would have the physician focus most of his/her energy and interest there instead of on tests. And rightly so.

Practically speaking, medical schools don't do well at teaching their charges History Taking and Physical Examination. With only a few hours of modest supervision, that class is generally given much less time than it is obviously due. "You will pick up the fine points of History and Examination in the hospital and in the clinics."

Amazingly, medical students spend MUCH more time poring over human corpses in anatomy lab than they do learning how to examine living humans. Thus, many medics are much more comfortable around dead, anesthetized or sedated patients than around live ones.

Physicians clearly need to be comfortable around a human body. And to be comfortable around a human body, a physician must be comfortable around human beings. And to be comfortable around human beings, a physician has to be comfortable with him/herself. None of these are requirements to graduate from medical school.

• Record keeping is notoriously poor - from the top down. That despite or maybe because of the volumes and volumes of charts and reports, documents and letters which pass through medical offices.

Here are some of the reasons:

1) Physicians commonly have poor handwriting. They scribble a lot. Some have miniscule scrawls. Legibility in writing is not a qualification for medical advancement.

I'm reminded of the story of a rich patient who sent an invitation to her physician to attend one of her holiday parties with an RSVP appended to it. The physician got the invitation in his office and read it between seeing patients. He decided to respond immediately rather than put it off.

Doctor scribbled his RSVP on a prescription slip, stuffed it in an envelope, and put the envelope in the outbox. The hostess was pleased to get "Doctor's note," but sadly couldn't read his writing. She was too embarrassed to call the office, so she went to her pharmacist. She just figured if anyone could read the doctor's handwriting, it would be a druggist.

After arriving at the drugstore, the lady stepped to the counter and stuck out the doctor's reply, saying, "I wonder if you can help me with this?" Before she had the chance to explain, the busy pharmacist wheeled around. He squinted and adjusted his glasses to the light. Then, he walked to the back of the shoppe.

The woman wondered what the drug man might be doing and was concerned that she hadn't been given time to explain. But within a few minutes, he was back with a bottle in his hand which he presented to the woman. He told her, "This should do the trick. Just go over to the cashier and she will take your money. Thank you."

2) Dictated and transcribed reports are more and more common now. But, many physicians dislike dictating and leave that job until forced to comply. The longer it takes to get reports completed, the more likely there will be lapses in memory and subsequent errors.

3) Physicians commonly repeat tests done by other physicians and other facilities because it takes time and trouble to track them down. And because doing the test in-house puts more money in the till. Either way, more forms and paper get added to charts. More papers to collect and organize, more papers to get misfiled.

4) File clerks make mistakes. The alphabet is easy to follow, in theory. But not always in practice.

5) Medical offices go through office workers frequently. Lack of continuity creates problems as in any office.

6) People move so much these days. Unless they keep track of their own records, much information easily can be lost over the years.

The inefficiencies of medical practice and the redundancies and errors in medical records are well known. Record keeping by computer is meant to remedy that situation. Hopefully it will, but probably to a limited degree. Many solutions create more problems. One thing it won't remedy is the reading of medical records which is a bit like your Congressman reading the laws that they enact. 2000-page laws rarely get read. Voluminous charts, whether they are manually or digitally (by computer) collated, are similar.

Only the top few pages generally get viewed along with relevant reports which are usually stuck in the back of the document.

Hospital Time

These days, newer hospitals are examples of extremes and extravagance, plastic and parquet, sterility and spotlessness. It used to be that people donated and bequeathed of their wealth to churches and related charities. Now, much of those monies go to building the new cathedrals of medicine.

The general public no longer believes that Jesus will save them from disease and death. But just maybe, "That shiny medical center they're building will pull us through serious sickness and keep us living for a long time."

Yet, there seems little justification for common reverence as to the abilities of Big Medicine and High Hospitals. Oh, the mystique is there. The white coats, the gloves and gowns, the speed and glamor, life and death moments. Stethoscopes and proctoscopes. Tubes and tethers which seem to channel life between patient and machines. It is, from some angles, mind-boggling. From others, smoke and mirrors and mirage.

Most of medical monies pass through hospitals, for treatment and care in the last weeks and months of people's lives. The addendum which is rarely added is that most of that care and those monies goes for nought. Diseases progress, people die pretty much on schedule - with or without medical care.

Actually, people may die at a faster rate with than without. A number of studies have been done over the years which compared death rates in hospitals during strikes versus typical periods when medics were on duty. In the 70s in Jerusalem, Bogota, and Los Angeles, there were dramatic decreases in the numbers of deaths during hospital and physician strikes. In other words, more people die in hospitals under "normal" conditions than when doctors are not at work. What might that tell you?

I have to admit that at one time I practically loved to work in the hospital. It was so busy. Something new around every corner. Another patient, a different disease or injury.

My early years in medicine were largely spent in emergency situations. The ER gladly gave the impression of patching people up and getting them back home, helping those in grave distress, saving lives. For a time, I swallowed the picture whole.

As I worked in other hospital deparments, I was given the opportunity to "peek inside" patient problems. Thinking that the mysteries would be there revealed. Secrets stripped bare.

Not so. At least in the vast majority of instances. There were only modest numbers of "real" successes. And sometimes, I even wondered about those. The hospital episode was only a small part of the whole drama.

Over time, I realized that along with the supposed wonders of the hospital came so many drawbacks which often made it seem like it should be "the last place to go when you're sick." Norman Cousins's story was current at the time and it helped solidify that thinking for me.

Cousins, then respected editor of the Saturday Evening Post, was diagnosed with ankylosing spondylitis (see In the Name of ...), was hospitalized and tested, and so on. After suffering with hospital procedures, he decided he could do better than the hospital and the usual medical routine as well as dispense with its intrusions into the healing process he desired. "I had a fast-growing suspicion that a hospital was no place for a person who was seriously ill. The surprising lack of respect for basic sanitation, the rapidity with which staphylococci and other pathogenic organisms can run through an entire hospital, the extensive and sometimes promiscuous use of Xray equipment, the seemingly indiscriminate administration of tranquilizers and powerful painkillers, more for the convenience of hospital staff in managing patients than for therapeutic needs, and the regularity with which hospital routine takes precedence over the rest requirements of the patient (slumber, when it comes for an ill person, is an uncommon blessing and is not to be wantonly interrupted) -- all these and other practices seemed to me to be critical shortcomings of the modern hospital. Perhaps the hospital's most serious failure was in the area of nutrition." (*Anatomy of an Illness*)

With his physician's approval, Cousins checked out of the hospital and into a hotel saving considerable money along the way. He took massive doses of Vitamin C (ascorbic acid) and dispensed with most medications while avoiding hospital indignities. Norman also gathered together an assortment of Hollywood and New York's funniest films and TV shows, most notably Marx Brothers movies and Candid Camera episodes. He found that "ten minutes of laughter had an anesthetic effect and would give me at least two hours of pain-free sleep."

Mr. Cousins treated himself to gradual recovery from a practically incurable disease. His personal physician had told him the odds were 1 in 500. His specialist had never seen a patient recover from the condition.

Everybody has stories about their hospital experiences. Some are uplifting and have happy outcomes. Many more are otherwise. The One Third Rule of Hippocrates holds as much for hospitals as general medical encounters. 1/3 get better, 1/3 stay the same, and 1/3 depart the hospital worse for the ordeal and expense.

The exact words of Hippocrates read as follows: "One third of patients can't be helped, another third get better without help, and the other third are suited for active and also potentially harmful medical treatment."

That thought reminds me that engaging the professional services of hospital or physician is one of the few modern situations where the patient gets absolutely no guarantee. Neither hospitals nor physicians guarantee anything.

A Money Back Guarantee is unheard of. If a mistake is made, the patient pays for the error as well as for things being made right. Even if it is for the removal of the wrong organ or appendage.

That kind of arrangement only goes in the medical system. Modern capitalism allows it nowhere else. How long would your automobile mechanic stay in business if he worked as physicians and hospitals do? How is it that patients and public are so accepting of such medical practices?

Here are some obvious problems with modern hospital care:

- The hospital (and clinic) is one of the rare businesses where you generally only find out the cost after your contract is completed. You often can't even get an estimate. Only the professionals know the codes for their services. And sometimes that is questionable.

You, the patient, don't get an estimate. Not unless, YOU bring the idea up. That happens rarely and is often taken as an affront. Such a question is somehow generally deemed as inappropriate in a "professional setting."

- Like the clinic, the hospital runs on its schedule. Not the patient's. Getting tests and procedures performed, vital signs taken, meals passed out and the dishes stowed away generally outrank patient comfort and concern. Then, there's the paperwork to document what has been done.

"Since there are so many patients to care for, we have to do it this way." Maybe medicine would do better with smaller hospitals. But, that would eliminate the high tech expensive machines which physicians and patients now think are indispensable to high quality medical care.

- Hospitals are institutions, run more and more to make money rather than to serve the public. Even not-for-profit hospitals "watch the bottom line" very closely. There is a constant battle between income and care. The latter loses by default often before the options are surveyed.

The days of physician as Hospital President (CEO) are over. At the top of the modern hospital hierarchy stands a business person, the hospital administrator, who has studied a lot more about finances and marketing than health or disease. S/he has been tapped to keep the institution visible to the public, to sustain a fluid and profitable operation and to provide the "highest quality medical care possible." The order of priority as written above should be considered accurate.

In defense of most any hospital administrator, s/he surely has the hardest job in the hospital. Hospitals and their administration are easy targets. There is always something going wrong if for no other reason than they are crystallized institutions with little flexibility. And the administrator bears the brunt of criticism coming from staff physicians, other medical workers, patients, the public in general and the media.

- The hospital is a "Hurry Up and Wait" sort of place. Things go from emergent to a standstill in a moment. How many people have I heard say, "They told me it was urgent that I get to the hospital to be admitted. Then, I sat through the weekend waiting for something to happen. I should have gotten up and left."

"Hurry Up and Wait" describes much of medical practice where some symptom or medical finding calls for rapid evaluation and intended treatment. Appointments are made quickly, testing is hurriedly done. Then, there is almost always a waiting period to "get all the results back" before proceeding.

Physicians and hospitals alone are certainly not responsible for this state of affairs. A friend recently emailed me that her 20-something daughter had told her about a breast lump she had discovered. The mother raced her to an emergency room which started the ball rolling. A week later, the two went to their usual physician. But, the tests of the previous week had not been read or the reports not transmitted through some glitch in the system. The scenario went on for weeks with the suggestion that "we should just follow the lump on a regular basis."

The mother, you might expect, was concerned and anxious. What she had considered to be an emergency had turned out to be routine and drawn out in the medical system.

"Shouldn't she have been upset and protested about the delays and attitude of the system?" you might ask. Probably not for two reasons. The mother is a nurse with decades of experience and she knows what a Real Emergency is. The daughter had been aware of the breast lump for three months before she told her mother.

- Theoretically, nothing is supposed to happen in the hospital without *doctor's orders*. Even an aspirin requires an order. And, be sure, you will pay well for that one aspirin.

I have been quite fortunate to have spent only a bare few days in my life in a hospital bed. The first two were when I was a child and due to relatively minor injuries.

The third time occurred during my 89-year-old father's latter days. He already had been in the hospital for a few days when his chest had filled with fluid which was drained. Later, his physician required him (my father never would have objected) to go back to the hospital for more tests and a biopsy to determine if he had cancer, which was suspected and almost certain to be found. (I wonder what Dr. Smythe would have said about the scenario.)

Dad had to spend more days in the hospital than he had anticipated. Finally, he was to be discharged on the following day. But, he had gotten a case of cabin fever, "I want to go home now." Still, the consensus ruled that he should remain in the hospital until the next morning.

When all else failed, I decided to stay overnight and keep Dad company in his two-bedded room. I napped and he napped. But, he woke again and again having chest discomfort. I asked the nurse for some Tylenol. "I will take them to him," I said.

"No. I will have to administer them myself. But first, I will have to see if we have a *doctor's order* for them."

The Tylenol did nothing. He had been using a heating pad at home to make himself comfortable. "That should be easy."

I returned to the nurses' station. "My father would like to try a heating pad. Can we get one for him?"

"Well, I don't know seeing the lateness of the hour. I will have to get a *doctor's order*. And you will have to pay for it."

Really? Is there anything free in the hospital, other than air and water? Maybe not even water, these days.

When the morning finally came and Dad was finally resting a bit, a phlebotomist (blood drawer) came in to take "more blood." I put my foot down. He was resting and going home in a few hours. Hospital routine!

- "There they are, again! All those sick people. Lots more of them in the hospital than at the clinic. And they seem a whole lot sicker. Only they are kind of spread out in double and single rooms and hidden from the rest, most of the time. A number of the hospital staff look more like patients than "health care workers."

Hospitals are about sickness. They are invested in sickness and cater to the sick. If you really want to be well, hang out with healthy people in healthy environs.

Courthouses concentrate legal powers. Prisons and jails collect criminal forces. Those forces are dominant, whatever the warden says. Hospitals contain whirlpools of disease energies, some of them more malignant than others. Which helps explain the next problem associated with a hospital, however hard it tries to fulfill its medical mission.

- The hospital is the Center of Iatrogenic Illness. All medical centers create lots of disease and injury. Disease breeds more disease. Trauma and violence attract surgical intervention and sequelae.

Iatrogenic (physician-caused) disease is a major concern in most any medical facility. Intervening in the human body and the life process - diseased or otherwise - often produces negative, damaging and sometimes deadly results. Some of those results happen due to the nature of medicine and others because of error.

Everyone makes mistakes. I am sure I made my share when practicing medicine. Mine were likely more of omission than commission. Fortunately, most of my "mistakes" were intentional and - I thought - modest deviations from standard practice.

I was particularly close to one incident back in my family practice internship days which may give the reader an idea about how "stuff happens," even in hospitals. It occurred shortly after I left the Internal Medicine Service. I had been following Mrs. Kathleen Morton for several days. Kathleen, the wife of an active-duty officer, was an attractive, introverted woman in her early forties, who had originally been admitted to the psychiatric ward because of a depressive episode.

Suddenly, she developed a pulmonary embolus and was transferred to the intensive care unit, where Dr. Alexander, my supervisor, and I managed her care. We gave her pain relievers and IV blood thinner, standard for such a problem. A complication of the embolus soon developed: a one-sided pleural effusion (fluid in the chest cavity outside the lung). Alexander said, "Let's wait a few days. Her body will resorb it soon enough."

The effusion was relatively small in size, but showed no signs of dissipating on its own. We waited a few more days after she was moved from intensive care to the ward, checking the status of the effusion with portable chest Xrays.

When the effusion still wouldn't budge, Dr. Alexander decided that a tube had to be inserted to drain the fluid sitting in her chest cavity. I was still in no hurry to add another trauma to Mrs. Morton's body. Despite what the Xray showed, Morton seemed to be doing reasonably well. And Alexander and I couldn't connect during the final days of my stint to perform the bedside procedure. Besides, I was never much into invasive procedures and I didn't enjoy being around the Attending Physician.

All in all, I was relieved when the end of my watch arrived without the chest tube insertion having occurred. I turned over my patients including Mrs. Morton to the new intern team of Drs. Joe Handsome and Jon Stone. Joe and Jon were the most aggressive and energetic of the whole first-year resident group. They jumped into that internal medicine rotation at a running pace.

Immediately, they decided to "get things moving" on the ward. And that included inserting Mrs. Morton's chest tube. They got Dr. Alexander's okay and reviewed Mrs. M.'s chart and Xrays. Joe and Jon set up for what was anticipated to be a quick and simple 1-2-3 procedure.

Unfortunately, the "guys" made a mistake. From a distance, the error is almost unfathomable. But, it happened as such things are wont to occur in the "healing" arts. The new teammates inserted the tube into the wrong chest cavity. Instead of relieving a minor problem, they created a new one. The chest tube had to remain in place for a time because the puncture caused a pneumothorax (air in the chest cavity) on Mrs. Morton's "good side." Joe and Jon had to go back, I imagine in sheepish chagrin, to insert a second tube on the correct side on another day.

Mistakes happen everywhere. Errors occur regularly in the hospital and in medicine with many untoward results. Regardless, "doing time" in a hospital may not be good for your health.

Pen Light

The author believes that far too much of medicine in the modern era has far too little to do with human beings, relationships and interactions. The medical stage is "lit up" by science and technology such that that portion of society has taken almost dictatorial control. Sometimes, results have been laudable. Often, the outcomes have been dubious.

A favorite story tells about the 13th century mystic, Jallaludin Rumi, who was known to use unusual teaching methods to get his message across. One day, a student quietly entered his house to find the teacher crawling on his hands and knees. Rumi was then determinedly searching for something. The student watched for a time, not realizing that Rumi was quite aware he was in the room. Eventually, the student tired and asked, "Master, for what are you looking so diligently and so unsuccessfully?"

"My key. Come and help me," Rumi responded.

The student joined him in the search in a corner of the room near a window. But, he again tired of hunting for the key and asked, "Master, we have been looking for a long time here and have found nothing. Tell me more. How did you happen to lose the key? What were you doing when it happened? Do you recall?"

Rumi said, "Oh, yes. I was busy on the other side of the room at the bookcase when I found my key was missing."

The student piped up showing some frustration, "Then, why are we looking over here since you seem to have lost the key on the other side of the room?"

"Well, my son, because the light is better over here."

This story can be applied in many different situations. It most certainly fits the state of modern medical research and practices. Medicine, like most modern disciplines, focuses its energy understandably where the LIGHT is or seems to be better. Or, maybe where it points its instruments - eyes, scopes and machinery.

Physicians are known for their scopes. With few exceptions like a stethoscope, these implements have lights at the end of them. Such as otoscope, ophthalmoscope, endoscope, bronchoscope, anuscope, proctoscope, colonoscope, culposcope, cystoscope, arthroscope, laparoscope, etc. Practically every orifice - and then some - of the human body has a scope devoted to it.

Then, there is the plain old pen light. It apparently doesn't deserve to be called a scope because it is too small, cheap to manufacture and readily distributed as a freebie by drug company and other reps. The pen light is a physician's ever ready tool, handily kept in a coat or shirt pocket, and seemingly useful for "shining light," modest as it is in or on small spaces. Usually the mouth or nostrils.

Since it is practically ubiquitous and carried by most physicians, it seems to be an appropriate symbol for modern medicine. White coats and gloves, Xrays and blood tubes, pills and scalpels - and the Pen Light tell much of the story of the state of medicine. Future centuries will surely have different symbols to represent "a more enLIGHTened era."

The place of greatest apparent LIGHT varies with time. But for many generations now, the light has shined on the physical body, and thence to blood tests and Xrays and more recent innovations. Which fit neatly with the use of drugs and surgery. The Pen Light makes an appropriate symbol because it, like modern medicine, shines light on the surface of things, especially the physical form.

In past eras, medical practice focused on spirits, humors, and temperaments; bloodletting, purging, and cauterization. Even in this century, curing practices vary according to country and tradition. Curanderos, shamans, herbalists, psychics and other healers may well outnumber university trained physicians on a worldwide basis. Those practitioners look for LIGHT that shines for them in quite different areas. Likewise, psychosomatic medicine (a small, little-noticed field), Christian Science and New Thought try to shine the LIGHT differently to look for and respond to emotional, mental and spiritual causes and influences.

All western schools of medicine base themselves largely on the forms through which they treat. Chiropractic and osteopathy use hands on adjustments and manipulations, naturopathy - natural remedies. Acupuncture utilizes needles. Standard medicine (allopathy) uses treatments which directly oppose the effects of illness with powerful drugs and operations. In all these cases, the LIGHT is largely pointed at the physical body with regard to its ailments and its relief.

But to those who have eyes to see, it should become clear that Light is not just a physical phenomenon. The great scientist Albert Einstein hinted at this most provocatively when he said, "For the rest of my life I will reflect on what light is." (1919)

The mystical teacher Rumi was surely hinting that our searches - in medicine and otherwise - should go beyond the superficial routes of investigation. While common things are commonly found, their sources are not necessarily quite so obvious.

Many years ago, I heard another seemingly wise teacher speak at a medical symposium in Wichita, Kansas. Dr. Denis Burkitt was a well-traveled and experienced English surgeon who had long practiced his profession in Kenya and Uganda before he returned to his home country in the 1960s.

He had become famous initially for studying an unusual tumor found among African children which since bears his name as Burkitt's lymphoma. By the time I heard him speak, he was a force in western medicine because he had taken time to reflect on the differences in diseases found in civilized and primitive countries.

He cheerily told us that during his twenty years in Africa he had only removed the gall bladders of three patients (such surgery is very common in Europe and America) and two thirds of them (to be mathematical about it) had been royalty: African Queens. Burkitt went on to suggest - with charts, statistics, and commentary - that he believed that many diseases (including those of the gall bladder) of western civilization were due to the lack of fiber in the diet. Dietary fiber, bran, Metamucil, etc. got a big boost from Dr. Burkitt.

One slide he offered graphically (and humorously) suggested that Africans have few and small hospitals because they have many and large stools as a result of their high fiber diets. Westerners have few and small stools (because of diet) and thus many and large hospitals.

He showed another slide trying to make the analogy between a surgeon and a maintenance man. A sink is overflowing its confines and the Maintaining Surgeon is keeping his end up by catching the drips with big buckets and swabbing the deck - using surgical operations. The proper approach was, according to Dr. Burkitt, to unplug the sink - by addressing the causes of disease, some of them due to western diet.

Well, there was a further remedy. That was to turn the water off at the spigot. This metaphor adds an extra layer or two to Rumi's perspective. The LIGHT can be shined on the overflowing water, the plugged sink or the open spigot.

A Frugal Physician doesn't have to be a surgeon to get the bright idea that things are not always as simple as they seem on the surface. S/he might even take some time to hunt for the spigot. S/he takes the hint and realizes there are many dimensions which the naked eye does not see but undoubtedly affect human health and well-being. S/he is willing to search beyond the surface of patient bodies and self to discover deeper dimensions and more LIGHT.

Germs and Disease

Medicine spends almost all of its time attending, studying, testing, manipulating, medicating, and operating on the human body. Devoting so much time, energy and money is akin to worship. Clinics and hospitals might not unjustly be called Churches of the Body. Physicians, then priests thereof.

The next layer of the medical dilemma seems to be a somewhat similar reverence to the relatively hidden world of germs. Oh, how we love to fear them. Bernard Dixon, in his book entitled *Powers Unseen*, says, "Always, microbes lie in wait as opportunists, ready to exploit any *change in human behaviour or living environment*. Microbes, not macrobes, rule the world." (Note *italics* above.)

Still, we are not vanquished. There is hope. Real LIGHT at the end of a long tunnel of experience. Limited and shortsighted though it be, modern medical practice is slowly - very slowly - drawing us toward a broader understanding of disease and healing. The passion of physicians and researchers for microbes hints that doors will eventually open toward real LIGHT on the subject of things that are now quite hidden even from microscopes. In the meantime . . .

"Germs cause disease." That idea is akin to the modern belief in evolution. While there is some truth to both, there are large holes in each widely held hypothesis. The whole story is still out on Germ Theory and Darwinian Evolution.

Yes, I heard, "Germs cause disease." Every child knows this long-held, concise and supposed fact. Many learn it before they go to school. The idea is driven into us day in and day out on TV, in the newspapers, by friends and neighbors. We are impressed to gargle Listerine, sanitize the bathroom, sterilize our dishes, take antibiotics prophylactically, etc.

I had a significant problem with that idea from early on in my medical training - even before medical school. I remember sitting in my crude medical aid station in the boondocks of Vietnam in 1968-69. I often had time on my hands and spent many hours reading and trying to make sense of the Merck Manual of Diagnosis and Therapy. It was a compact book crammed with fine print which seemed to say that most every illness or syndrome known to medicine could be caused by one microbe or another.

As in many disciplines in the modern age, "Things are complicated." And so was and is disease and medical practice. There were lists and lists and more lists of causative agents for this or that problem. And germs were almost always high among them.

After I completed college with a degree in Medical Technology, I took my first and only job in that field in hospital bacteriology. Ouch! I lasted just a few months and went back to emergency room nursing until I arrived at medical school. While working in the Bacteriology Department, we spent our time pursuing, culturing and plating bacteria. Hoping to find something to treat with the growing arsenal of antibiotics.

We not only tested human beings for bacteria but regularly cultured inanimate objects as well. Weekly, one of the three of us in the department had to go around the hospital wards and swab the floors. That's right we took large cotton Qtips, ran them across the footpaths of the hospital, and then stuck the swabs in individual tubes of nutrient broth.

Before long we plated the cultures to see what kind of bacteria were collecting on our floors. They might be potential sources of contamination! At the time, carpets in hospitals were unthinkable because they could become hosts for even more of the ubiquitous microscopic critters!

Culturing the floor was practically the same as taking a swab to the streets or yards in the vicinity. Anything and everything there would certainly end up underfoot in the hospital. We made our regular "floor reports," but who cared? I suspect the reports were filed for inspection purposes.

I quickly tired of chasing bugs. That experience might well have given me a clue about challenges and headaches I would have in coming years with the "germ theory." Germs have been in vogue and blamed for practically every bad thing under the sun since the days of Pasteur and Koch. In many ways, evil germs took over where miasmas, humors, and spirits left off in the Middle Ages.

Germs were one of several things in my craw when I made an appointment during my second year to speak with the dean of the medical school, Dr. Robert Tuttle. This was before I started working on the wards and encountered Dr. Kirkendall. I basically told Dean Tuttle that, "I don't quite believe a lot of what they are teaching us in the academic end of school. I am having trouble swallowing all of it."

I didn't have the gumption to make it clear that I didn't believe in the prevailing germ theory because I knew Dr. Tuttle had been a professor of immunology and microbiology at Bowman-Gray School of Medicine prior to becoming Dean at UTMSH.

Tuttle listened gently without taking the slightest offense. Then, he talked to the tune of, "Our job is to teach medicine as we now understand it. It's surely far from perfect and continues to change frequently. Your job is to learn what we teach you. When you graduate and are on your own you will have some leeway on how you practice according to your own beliefs and understandings. Just go out and do what is expected of you and do it well. Your own time and opportunity will come soon enough."

I listened and tried for a time. But, my own ideas and mouth got in the way soon enough. My ideas about germs were just some of the stumbling blocks along the way. I know I was an exceptional case in med school. My compatriots ate the traditional medical meal, chewed on it happily while relishing the flavor.

Most physicians as well as the general public take it as established and irrefutable fact that germs cause disease. The idea is pretty much Gospel and influences so much of our behavior that to question it may seem sacrilegious. But, that hasn't held me back in the past and won't now.

"Germs do not cause disease," I say. "They can be a part of the picture, but are neither the biggest nor most important."

"Prove it," you might say. Well, I can't prove it any more than medical people can prove the usual belief. Medics do have lots of tests and research to support their case, but their conclusions are subject to challenge. As for me, I ask that we try to use some common sense as we take another look at common beliefs.

To begin, the world and our physical bodies are hosts to uncountable numbers of bacteria, viruses, fungi and the like. (Germs in other words.) Many of these are said to "cause disease." But, a thoughtful and economical physician might ask, "If these creatures are always with us, around us, and in us, how is it that we seem generally undiseased and healthy, and are not overwhelmed regularly by such microbial vermin? Explain that, please."

It is quite clear that microbes rarely cause us harm, and more often than not are helpful to us. We live in a state of comfortable coexistence with them and we have many cooperative relationships with these microscopic creatures. We give them a place to live and they help us synthesize vitamins, break down foodstuffs, and eliminate waste products. Most of this action occurs, but is not confined to, within the intestinal system.

Microbes also have functions that support the health of our skin and hair as well. All of their helpful chores are likely not yet discovered. This is simply the case because scientists have been pointing their lights in the other directions, hunting for "those disease makers."

One of their main tasks - as they fill an incredibly important niche in nature - is to aid in decomposition of dead, morbid, necrotic material wherever it may be found. Without the fulfillment of that function life would be impossible.

A basic premise which medicine largely ignores is that only when something goes wrong in our personal environment (see Dixon quote at begining of chapter) do bacteria seem to cause us harm, or at least make themselves more visible. Sometimes they just appear to cause harm or we imagine that they do. Bacteria and viruses have become "the usual and regular suspects." They take the wrap for practically every human ill, and come out looking much like evil personified. Though they are tiny, tiny microscopic fellows.

The influential 19th century chemist, Claude Bernard, said, "The seeds of disease are everywhere to be found. Whether they take root depends on the terrain on which they land." Thus came the idea of the "terrain factor," which gets too little attention in medical circles and the society in general. And, it may be even that seeds are not the best analogy for germs as they are seen producing disease. Too often it seems that microbes are "accessories after the fact" in the crimes we call disease.

Many germs are opportunistic like weeds. They say, "Weeds are a gardener's best critics." They take over terrain which is not well tended. The real problem in that case is not the weed, but the gardener. In a like manner, in human disease the real problem is rarely a microbe but the state of the affected individual and his/her environment. If we take a look at some of the most common "contagious" diseases, past and present, we can understand the points of view of Claude Bernard and others of his ilk.

Who is most likely to come down with influenza? Which people are at the top of the list to be given flu vaccine every year? What groups of people are most likely to become infected with West Nile Virus or SARS or Legionnaire's Disease? Who is most susceptible to E. coli diarrhea? Historically, who was most likely to succumb to tuberculosis, leprosy, malaria and tropical diseases?

The answer to all these questions is older, debilitated, already diseased or injured people. Secondarily, it is the malnourished, the stressed and anxious, the injured and maimed and hopeless. The hale and hearty, vital and virile, active and energetic need worry little about any of these contagious diseases unless confined to the trenches and terrors of war, the filth and rot of dying societies.

On the other side of the world, we see contagion affecting poor, starving and often war-ravaged civilian populations. In this case, many who become diseased are young but not robust for simple lack of adequate food and proper hygiene, for living in the dirt and being tormented by fear and trauma.

The medical profession has taken credit for increased lifespan and greater well-being in many populations because of vaccination and antibiotics. But, real credit is largely due to improvements in sanitation and hygiene, better housing, plentiful food, and overall improved living conditions in most parts of the world.

Despite the general rap and hype which is so common, germs are not king of the mountain, barbarian invaders standing at the gate waiting for opportune moments to kill. They are not predators, but generally more scavengers, feeders, members of the cleanup crew.

A Frugal Physician is careful about patting him/herself on the back because s/he might soon have to take the blame. In a similar way, let's not point the finger at the tiniest of creatures for problems which we create.

Germs are not our major nemeses. We surely are our own worst enemies. A Wise Doctor knows that and so should we all.

The Life That Lives on Man

Pondering on microbes brings to mind two more medical school professors. They stood out because of their specialty more than for their teaching abilities. The first got my fellow students' attention, the second even got mine at least on one occasion.

Dr. Herbert DuPont was our new Chief of the Department of Infectious Disease. Tall and young, blond and bright, he was also out to "slay the dragons," which in those and these days are quite paradoxically tiny, tiny microbes.

Regardless, there is some sort of glamor even into the present day which holds over from when Pasteur and Lister and Koch and others began to supposedly "stop germs in their tracks." Whatever DuPont spewed forth in lectures, my fellows ate it up. I had "been there, done that," and was hardly impressed. Humans are bigger than bugs, however you stack things up.

I recall that DuPont was becoming famous at the time for his elixir used for treating Montezuma's Revenge, South American dysentery, which everyone imagines is assuredly due to food and water contaminated by bacteria. Interestingly, his treatment was common, plain old PeptoBismol - pepsin and milk of bismuth. A bit of a surprise.

Dr. Richard Conklin was a lecturer (rather THE lecturer) in Virology. He taught the whole course. From the very first class, I remember him bemoaning the grand importance of viruses in modern medicine. And the sad state of affairs in which he was only given a paltry twenty hours to teach us the fine points of virology. That said, "I will try to keep my lectures brief and get you out well before the end of the each class period!"

Conklin had another profession prior to medicine and joining the faculty of UTMSH. He had been a whale pathologist. During the last period of our Virology course, he gave us a slide show of the Orcas.

I remember that session being one of the few high points of medical school studies. Paradoxical as it was. Probably the best hour-long presentation in the whole of my medical school career was not on human beings, or even health and disease, but on whales! Whales, humans and microbes all play their roles in the Big Screen of Life. None of the above "Rules the World." But, all have important parts to play.

Those tiny creatures called germs have necessary and important functions. Even in and on your body and mine. Common sense suggests that we learn to accept what is - even germs.

We can learn many things from bacteria. That we are not alone, that much has been hidden from us over the ages, and that much more is left to be brought to our awareness in the course of time and evolution. Microbes were largely unknown until 150 years ago - along with a host of other scientific matter. What other worlds and creatures are yet to be recognized in and around us?

Science and technology may have brought us much wealth and opportunity in the material world, but undoubtedly there are more dimensions of existence to be explored. While we have harnessed fire and electricity and nuclear energy to our uses, we still know not their source and full potential. Just like our own.

We still generally just understand the topmost layers of things. We count and categorize, identify and name, examine and investigate many things as yet coming to limited understandings because we still shine our LIGHT on the surface. The life and meaning of most parts of nature and our very own selves remain to be uncovered. The world and our own beings are like onions. Layer wrapped upon layer and all of them practically inseparable. Many are quite invisible.

As a matter of fact, we still don't understand the most prominent part of human anatomy all that well: Our skin which is the natural home to billions and billions of microbes. "The horrid truth is that each of us has about as many bacteria and yeasts on the surface of his or her skin as there are people on earth; far from being 'clean' after a bath the number of organisms released from the surface actually goes up as they emerge from the nooks and skinny crannies where they multiply." (Michael Andrews)

"They're everywhere." The fact that germs are everywhere and practically immune to being dislodged from their perches scares many people, the medical profession in particular. Medics and the media spread the word and create phobia - germophobia - of our tiny fellow travelers. Often, fear of little germs produces more problems than the reality of things. Because, in fact, their presence is usually quiet and unobtrusive.

But, fear of bacteria has become quite common since they were discovered by the likes of scientist Louis Pasteur. Pasteur was one of the first to relate the presence of bacteria to disease. His hard work and researches brought him fame as well as a morbid fear of dirt and infection. Pasteur avoided the shaking hands for fear of being contaminated with the germs which made him well known. But, Dr. Louis may have overestimated those fellows. Like many moderns, he certainly overreacted to being up close and personal with them.

One of the major works of bacteria is cleaning up dying, decomposing matter. That is one of their favorite breeding grounds. Germs are a vital (note the irony) part of the decomposition process. Without their help, the world would be practically incapable of change, turnover and renewal. New life requires death. Death necessitates destruction and decomposition.

We need to get comfortable with the fact that, "Germs are just about everywhere." Often, as on human skin, they are neither parasites nor pathogens, but neighbors along for the ride. Borrowing our landscape while they clean up after us. We generally tolerate them quite well because they are "working with us."

When our "interior milieu" (Claude Bernard) is disturbed or threatened, microbes may become overgrown or even participate in our disease processes. Friendly germs can become otherwise when we don't keep up our end of shared housekeeping.

Skin is a miniature world of its own, as other parts of the human body, and has its own ecology. Microbes - our own flora and fauna work to produce a balanced state as long as we do.

Areas of human skin may normally have from hundreds to millions of bacteria per square inch of surface. When our skin is without disease or injury, these microbes stay in a healthy balance with over bodily coat.

Interestingly, no amount of scrubbing or scraping, iodizing or decontaminating will clear them away. A bath, shower or scrub actually raises the number of microbes released from our skins by as much as three hundred percent for up to ten hours. It is IMPOSSIBLE to sterilize the skin. A surgeon's ten-minute scrub generally brings more germs to the surface of the skin than it cleans away. This might make a thinking person question the value of the elaborate rituals which occur in operating rooms prior to surgery.

Curiously, scientific research has shown it to be almost impossible to create infections on the skin experimentally. All sorts of attempts have been made to produce them. But, short of injuring the skin and "pouring on the bugs," skin infections can't be created in the laboratory. That finding has significant implications. What does it suggest to the reader?

Bodily bacteria actually do us great service. In their brief lives (sometimes as little as twenty minutes), they digest dead organic material, not just on our skin but everywhere. As much of HALF of the waste matter which passes out of the large intestine in a bowel movement is composed of the remains of these very short-lived microscopic creatures.

But, what about the great plagues of past ages? Filth was clearly one of the main intermediaries of the plague, as much as medical people want to blame them on a tiny bacillus. The congestion within cities, terrible or nonexistent sanitation, general filth and RATS were major vectors of the plague and similar diseases which decimated millions during the Dark Ages. But, the rats were really like the weeds in the garden, the opportunists taking advantage of a good thing - for them.

I am reminded of a neighbor who left her house unattended for several months. I suspect it was also left less than spotless on her departure. She had had a number of cats and dogs in residence with her. When she returned, the mice had taken over. The owner couldn't move back in until things were cleaned up. She was quite upset with the little rodents. But, where do you think the real responsibility lay?

Without filth in the cities of dirty Europe, there would have been no plague. Without the rot and blight and fear in the front lines of World War I, there would have been no trench fever, typhus, and dysentery. In recent times, the cholera epidemic occurring after the earthquake in Portau Prince was largely due to overcrowding in tents, inadequate sanitation, fear and the effects of long-standing poverty in Haiti.

Those who study epidemics are apparently puzzled why there have been few recent outbreaks of such diseases. Common sense suggests that, while germs are still constantly all around us, the disease-producing conditions of filth and muck and rot are not as common and blatant as in past.

Nature created the microbial kingdoms to be part of the world ecology, as well as part of our own. Due to our own ignorance and arrogance, sloth and pride, we have tried to make them responsible for practically every ailment under the sun and under the skin. We have thus misrepresented and calumniated our little friends. We also have empowered them falsely to our own detriment.

Being relatively comfortable with the natural world, a Frugal Physician recognizes the necessary place of microbes in the world. S/he carefully considers and reconsiders blaming any disease on germs. So might you.

Bigger Bugs or Bigger People

From my experiences in hospital bacteriology, medical practice and day-to-day common sense living, I came to a perspective which is clearly at odds with the usual beliefs of medicine, the media and middle America. I am not alone, but in a small minority. It is clear to me that most people in western society are somewhere between cautious and downright petrified of microbes, bacteria, germs, bugs. We seem to have swung with the pendulum to the opposite extreme from that which held sway a few hundred years ago. When sanitation meant dumping chamber pots out the window into the streets below every morning. When people only came near water when forced to. When bathing was a monthly affair - sometimes yearly, sometimes just at birth and death. When the pores of the skin were meant to be guarded from intrusion and protected from water. When the populace cleaned their houses and linens, but not their bodies. Cleanliness and Godliness - at least in the western world had nothing in common.

Now, we have gone to the other extreme. And then some, because of technology and accepted science. In the medical arena as well as in homes and workplaces. At home, pantries and shelves are loaded with cleansers, antiseptics, deodorants, and disinfectants. We don't just clean and brush, we scrub and scour and rinse and repeat. If some cleaning is good, then more must be better.

The Centers for Disease Control (CDC) has become the federal government's watchdog to guard the public against bugs on the loose. In fact, like police departments, the CDC usually catches up to epidemics and disease outbreaks after the fact. The culprits are most always determined to be microbes, whether evidence and cases are clearly defined or not. I often wonder if propaganda doesn't outweigh proof in most instances.

In the hospital and clinic environment, bigger and bigger pushes have been made in recent years to protect one patient from the next, providers from patients, and patients from providers. We have moved from one extreme to the other in the course of 170 years.

The early impetus to get physicians and hospitals to "clean up their act" goes back to the 1840s when simple hand washing was forced upon medics and students in obstetrics and surgery. Ignaz Semmelweis was an astute physician who prevented childbed fever but challenged the norm of the medical profession. He brought change among his colleagues, but not without personal cost.

Semmelweis adopted the simple practice of handwashing with a chlorinated lime solution while working in Vienna General Hospital's First Obstetrical Clinic where the wards of doctors previously had three times the mortality of those of midwives. Women about to deliver begged to be attended by midwives of the Second Clinic knowing the bad reputation of the First. Physicians and medical students routinely shuffled from conducting autopsies to performing deliveries with cadaveric material on their hands.

Common sense certainly didn't rule in those days. Dirt and blood were as common as soap and water are now.

We often look over our shoulders and wonder, "How could they have lived that way? It's clear that they missed something. They believed spirits and humors caused their diseases. They just couldn't imagine the obvious."

Yet, ignorance marches on. In coming generations, those who follow us will look back and say, "Did they really give so much power to germs? How could they separate themselves from each other with gloves and masks and shields? They thought they were quite advanced, but did they really know much more than the barber-surgeons and potion makers of earlier centuries?"

The author is relieved that he doesn't work within the medical system in the 21st century. There are many reasons, chief among them being the mandated and constant use of plastic gloves. Gloves and safety precautions (along with other modern penchants for dispassion, medical-legal issues, time and paper work) make it harder for medical people to have real human contact with patients.

I look back and remember the time when I trained and worked as a medical technologist (lab tech). Morning blood draws were the routine.

We made the rounds bright and early. Knocked on doors, entered quietly into patient rooms. Presented ourselves as assigned to collect blood samples. Got our tubes and needles together. Put a rubber hose around the patient's arm, just above the elbow and waited until the antecubital vein bulged a bit. Swabbed it with an alcohol wipe, punctured the vein and let the blood flow. (Everyone knew that the swab was for looks only. It had no effect on germs whatsoever.)

We never used gloves. Actually, they would have and certainly do now interfere with the ability to feel and find a vein under the forefinger. Puncturing a vein is not always straightforward. Vessels don't always jump out even with a tourniquet and pumping of extremity muscles. Many times, veins have to be searched for, coaxed to appearance, encouraged to make their presence known. Even then on occasion, the vein can be missed or injured allowing blood to escape into surrounding tissue. The reader probably knows the result and may have wondered if the blood test was worth the hematoma.

Gloves get in the way in most any procedure - even surgery - or business. They do come in handy in many situations and are a means of real protection. But very often in the medical setting, gloves do not really protect, but rather intrude and set up barriers to gathering information and getting in touch with patients.

Physicians rarely get close to their patients. When they do touch them, it is almost always with gloves covering their hands and interceding between the two. Their practice being to prod and poke, invade and incise.

If we are really as advanced as we imagine, we should be able to find ways to reduce the distance between practitioner and patient. Rather than making for more distance except for disturbing intrusions. Can't we do any better?

But, the big bogey remains our belief in and terror of Almighty Germs. One might think that big, hairy and scary Microbe Armies are lurking at the gates of the city, approaching by unwatched thoroughfares, nearing our doorsteps with clear intention to "take us down."

Media-supported myths about the powers of bugs promote fears of "catching the flu," AIDS and other germ-borne diseases. "Those predators are out there stalking us constantly," so suggest the media and the medical community.

Remember Bernard Dixon (*Powers Unseen*): "Microbes rule the world." One might wonder for whom people like Mr. Dixon work. Does Dixon work for the medical-industrial complex or for living, breathing human beings?

Isn't this common nightmare much like those that have passed before in the guise of attacking spirits, evil forces, dark witches? In days of yore, priests and patriarchs said prayers, made the sign of the cross, performed safeguarding rituals to keep noxious forces at bay. Today, we use vaccines routinely, antibiotics indiscriminately, and back them up with potent propaganda and frequent testing. The physician's white jacket, mask and gloves, stethoscope (for those so concerned, stethoscopes most certainly are effective vectors for the spread of germs) and inscrutable rituals add to the forces arrayed against the microbial enemies.

Now, what is the real effect of such equipment, methods and ceremony? Do germs care or notice? Isn't the whole process adding to fear and creating problems instead of addressing real ones?

I, for one, hold a halfway original stance with regard to any microbial menace. Emulating a recent president, I say, "Bring 'em on. I'm bigger and tougher and smarter than any of you. It will take more than an army of you guys to do me any harm.

"As long as I have vitality, strength and integrity, I need have no fear of the likes of you. Let's continue as friends and co-workers. Peace, brothers."

Playing Catch

People readily accept most modern medical thinking, especially regarding germs and disease. In part, because they are relieved of responsibility. "I caught that nasty crud from who knows whom and got some antibiotics. The doctor says it's going around but I should be better in a few days."

The latter part of the statement is no doubt true. The perennial wisdom goes: "Get the flu and see the doctor, you'll be better in a week. Get the flu and stay home you'll recover in seven days." Those seven days can, however, feel longer than a week as you allow nature to do its work. Unaided and undisturbed. You are likely to become anxious and want to be better yesterday, not in seven days or even tomorrow.

We tend to think that any acute illness is contagious, dropped upon us by some sinister outside force. "They gave it to me. I was infected unknowingly." We believe ourselves to be innocent victims of blind malicious forces which are set loose in the world from time to time. They impregnate the unsuspecting and only the hallowed medical man can turn back the enemy.

With chronic illness, patients often but not always wonder, "How could it happen to me? What did I do to deserve this state of affairs?" The big problem common to many chronic diseases is that with or without medical care, "It ain't going away."

Fortunately, some people with long-term conditions get the message and learn from their dilemmas. They recognize their Disease does not have a lock on power and they can rest some of it back over time while growing through the experience.

But generally in acute and chronic disease, patients and physicians support the belief that the condition occurred unjustly. Bad things happening to good people. "The wrong guy got this disease but we will find a remedy for it and get you back to duty. Sooner the better."

But, really! In many cases, the "afflicted" is like a child in a candy store with a gumball in his mouth. His mother says, "Now, how did you get a hold of that?"

"I didn't take it. A stranger gave it to me. No, I think I found it on the floor. Honest."

Or like front page scandal sheet news, CELEBRITY CAUGHT WITH DRUGS BY POLICE. DENIES RESPONSIBILITY.

"Oh, officer. I don't know how those things got in my purse. Someone, I won't name names, must have put them there. I am innocent, I assure you." Methinks the lady protests too much.

Nonetheless, "catching disease" is an apt metaphor. It just requires a bit of contemplation to bring the idea into focus. To "catch" anything implies active participation. You don't catch a ball without sticking your hand out, often with a glove, and being open to receive - to catch.

If you know how to play catch, you can do it with one eye closed, etc. We catch disease often with one eye closed. More often with both of them closed. Still, it is an active, if unconscious process. Here is another way to look at it. In many ways, illness is like a gift. It has to be accepted, or it is not received. A gift you didn't ask for, but nonetheless needed.

This thinking opposes common belief: "Catching the flu (or other disease) is like an accident." Such a view suggests that illness and injury happen totally at random. Nature goes crazy. The world is without laws. And we are surrounded by the Wild Bunch.

If this were true, we most certainly would require even more physicians and gloves, drugs and vaccines than we now utilize. We all would be taking antibiotics continuously to protect against the next onslaught. If pathogenic germs are ever-present - waiting to invade and destroy, why don't we have more outbreaks and epidemics? Shouldn't they be constant?

The simple truth is that "Like attracts like." Illness and injury may result from mishaps and mistakes, but they are never truly accidental. Cause lies behind all things in the world, including disease. You can trust that your condition or problem suits you or you would not have been so blessed.

Disease and death affect us all because we are all mortal beings. They are part of the process, occur in some ordered fashion and have something to teach us and our physicians. If we pay attention. A Frugal Physician does.

What Do We Really Know?

The human race is both arrogant and ignorant at the same time. The medical profession as a whole may be justly described with the same words. Arrogance? They aren't called Medical Deities for nothing. At the same time consider the state of health of the public and the medical care system, which most everyone believes needs "fixing," and ignorance becomes a meaningful term.

We think we know so much, when actually we know so little. Like adolescents who think they know more than their parents. When they both are just blindly struggling along the way because neither have a road map for the journey. We are not far beyond the Biblical pronouncement which says, "If a blind man lead a blind man, they both fall in the ditch."

Not long ago (1997), scientific journalist John Horgan published a book called *The End Of Science: Facing The Limits Of Knowledge In The Twilight Of The Scientific Age*. Horgan believes all major scientific discoveries - natural selection, the double helix, the big bang, the relativity and quantum theories - have been made. Only refinements are left and no more revolutions or revelations are yet to be had. Just details.

Interestingly, my reading of history indicates that similar kinds of thinking were in vogue at the turn of the preceding two centuries. In any period, this seems like a foolish Know-It-All attitude. How arrogant to think that we have plumbed the width, breadth and depth of creation in the course of a few hundred years of scientific studies. By which we are just beginning to scratch the surface of understanding. This is most obvious when we consider how little we really know about our own bodies.

What do we know of the origins of life or even of the conception of a human being? How many secrets has the Earth yet to divulge? How little of the solar system - not to mention the galaxy - have we investigated in any meaningful way? And that just from purely materialistic standpoints. How many ills do we not in the least understand?

Dr. Lewis Thomas, a biologist, researcher, administrator and wise physician, hit the nail on the head when he wrote, "The only solid piece of scientific truth about which I feel totally confident is that we are profoundly ignorant about nature. [Humans are parts of nature, are they not?] Indeed, I regard this as the major discovery of the past hundred years of biology." (*The Medusa and the Snail*)

A Frugal Physician subscribes to the suggestion that, "The more we know, the less we know." With such perspective, we may be able to better place ourselves in the scheme of things. We are always just beginning the next leg of the journey, scientific or otherwise.

This attitude is not new, but rather reaches back to the ancients. "He who thinks he knows, doesn't know. He who knows he doesn't know, knows." Borrowing from the Tao Te Ching, Joseph Campbell (*The Power of Myth*) resurrected this pithy aphorism which might help us all consider our own limited mental abilities and understandings.

George Bernard Shaw said it a little differently. "He knows nothing and thinks he knows everything." GBS was probably speaking of an individual, but the quote might apply reasonably well to the whole human race.

My own mother put the idea into country vernacular. "He thinks he knows it all, but he really doesn't know his head from a hole in the ground." Sometimes, head was replaced by another part of human anatomy.

The expanses of inner and outer worlds - minute and vast, which we presently understand to only a relative degree, suggest that there are many realms yet to explore. They just won't look like the ones we have gotten used to. That is why many - even scientific "experts" - have not recognized them.

The future belongs to prudent people, Frugal Physicians, open-minded searchers and the likes of Albert Szent-Gyorgyi who said, "Discovery consists in seeing what everyone else has seen and thinking what no one else has thought."

To think that science has figured it all out in a span of a few centuries seems stupid as well as arrogant. We may have some handles on geology and astronomy and practical sciences, but we certainly have a long way to go to truly understand the human organism and life in general. We can use electricity and fire, but know not their true sources. We can count and name the planets and stars, but reckon not what keeps them on course. Or what it is that endlessly fuels the Sun, or raises a seed from the earth. On and on, the recitation can go.

We haven't even gotten used to the present horizons before they begin to change in front of us. There are many hidden implications of quantum physics and the microscopic worlds which we have yet to fathom.

Annie Dillard tells us *Even A Stone Can Teach*. If we are smart enough to pay attention to it. The simple premise is that learning opportunities are everywhere. People who live close to the land know this well. "Lift the stone and there you will find me. Split the wood and I am there." (*Gospel of Thomas*)

The color of the sky as the sun rises in the morning may have something to say to us. The flight of migratory birds surely has a message to offer. An abundance of bees or grasshoppers or porcupine or antelope in one year or season may give hints to us. I'm sure the list can be expanded almost endlessly.

Farmers and ranchers and naturalists and meteorologists learn much from such phenomena. Physicians and patients might do as well with the symptoms and feelings that we experience from time to time.

There is a flow and rhythm in the natural world which can be apprehended by paying attention to the sky and the water and the land and the animals upon it. So too, do we humans have our own observable rhythms and seasons of body and mind and feelings.

Too often, we just naively believe that we should feel happy and healthy and energetic and beautiful every day of every week of every month of every year of our lives. And if we don't, "Then, I'm sick. And that's bad. And I must get to feeling like normal soon or I'll have to go to the doctor and get him to make me feel better."

I remember over the years having a cold or flu or the like. A friend would say solicitously, "I'm so sorry that you feel bad. I sure hope you feel better right away."

I accepted the well-meaning sentiment. But, I more and more believe that aches and pains and colds and flus and the ague are just as much a part of life as happy or vital moments are.

Life is never without sorrow or pain. A fetus struggles to be born. A seedling strives in the dirt and mud and muck toward the light of the sun and the life of the spring.

Over the years, we have been brainwashed to think that we should always look trim, smell like Dial, smile with Crest, sound like a bell, and move like a model. If we don't, we better get cracking or go see the doctor.

Maybe so. But, maybe not. Accepting what is in the outer world and within ourselves is just as key to health as any medical checkup or examination. Probably more so.

Years ago, I went through a traumatic period during my family practice internship in Fort Benning, Georgia. I had been recently graduated and believed, although I was still in training, "I'm a doctor now. I should be able to prescribe according to my own lights and chosen methods." (Dean Tuttle had said I would be able to do that, but probably not as soon as I had in mind.)

Within a few weeks, I was placed on probation and scrutinized closely. And that was not the half of it. I became depressed and before my internship was over experienced (I won't say caught) hepatitis - inflammation of the liver. I turned yellow like a canary. I came to understand - that at least in my case - as the Chinese say, "The liver is the seat of smoldering anger." I was holding onto frustrations and resentment and fears instead of accepting things as they were and getting on with life.

I remember making rounds and looking over my shoulder imagining that someone was about to call me on the carpet. Or, cringing every time my number came up on the hospital paging system. "What did I do wrong now?"

At one point, I made a list of a dozen or so terms I used to express anger without using the word. Like fibbing isn't quite lying, I figured irritated or bothered or pissed off wasn't as unseemly as being plain old angry.

The learnings occurred over time and are far from complete. The liver has been quiescent and comfortable for years now. Not that I haven't had more lessons to learn and more aches and pains and injuries along the way.

The big - yet so simple - lesson I gathered from my internship travails came through one brief visit to a counselor in Atlanta. In the midst of an hour session, his simple statement, that I should "Go with the flow," hit home. I didn't immediately learn to regularly flow like a river, but I did begin to catch the rhythm of the current from time to time.

This is a Taoist view, like the one shared by Joseph Campbell. Learning to flow with the times and the seasons of our lives reminds me of the wonderful prayer: "God grant me the serenity to accept the things I can't change, the courage to change the things I can, and the wisdom to know the difference."

This prayer is really just good common sense and so is learning to "go with the flow." Wise people and physicians can make use of these understandings for the betterment of every one.

In the Name of . . .

Terminology is of key importance in medicine as it is now practiced. It goes hand in glove with diagnosis and labeling.

Regular physicians spend huge amounts of time, money and energy searching for names to put on problems, diagnoses to write on reports, labels to offer patients, codes to give to insurance companies.

They often think to themselves quietly or out loud, "We have to get to the bottom of this condition, make a diagnosis, so we can get treatment started." A sense of urgency to find a label may become as much a problem as the original presenting complaints.

Patients often add other layers to the drama by having to KNOW. "What have I got? Please tell me. Is it serious? I have to know what IT is. Soon. The waiting is just killing me."

Physicians sooner or later come up with a name, tag or label. After a string of tests, procedures, appointments, time and expense.

But, many labels and diagnoses are just hollow epithets. They have little or no substance because diseases - in the sense we generally think of them - do not exist. As Samuel Hahnemann said centuries ago, "There are no diseases, only sick people."

This is a hard one for physicians as well as patients to grasp. Physicians are so trained to work diligently to find some enemy to combat. "Investigate, identify, treat, cure."

Patients hope upon hope that first, "I don't have anything serious." Second, "If I got IT, I sure hope they have a silver bullet on hand."

Years ago, I sat down and made a list of categories for common diagnoses (diagnostic labels). This list and medical nomenclature in general make it quite clear that in the majority of illnesses, "We honestly don't know."

Unfortunately, patients don't understand medicalese. Doctors aren't as forthcoming as they might be. And they have to at least act as if they KNOW. Medical jargon and terminology help ease their insecurity.

The following is my latest, yet certainly incomplete, list of "We Don't Know" diagnoses. Still, it is more than twice as long as the earlier version.

1) Benign - as in prostatic hypertrophy. Not malignant, but neither do we know the cause.

2) Essential - as in hypertension. Essentially, the cause is not known.

3) Primary - as in tumor. Means the problem is not secondary to a detectable source.

4) Etiology Unknown - "We simply can't find the cause, but we are still looking."

5) Idiopathic - the same as etiology unknown. In his book *The Human Body*, Isaac Asimov commented on the term idiopathic he had found in the 20th edition of *Stedman's Medical Dictionary*: "A high-flown term to conceal ignorance."

6) Syndrome - as in autoimmune or wasting. Syndrome is generally a hodge podge of symptoms which is not defined well enough to be

called a disease.

7) Eponymous - as in Lou Gehrig's disease. Putting someone's name on a set of symptoms makes the condition more personal, but the cause usually remains unknown. Many of these conditions are also alternatively called syndromes, as in Sjogren's or Down's.

8) Stress-induced - pointing to mental-emotional influences. This is a common backup label used when a physical cause can't be found for the problem. Then, it can be blamed on the environment or on emotions. "Go see a psychiatrist."

9) Viral - so-called viral diseases can mimic all sorts of problems. But like bacteria, viruses are generally omnipresent and innocuous. "It seems to be an infection, but it's not bacterial. So, you must have a virus."

Viruses are blamed for everything these days. A friend told me how her mother was concerned about the granddaughter. "She better be careful spending so much time in front of that computer. She might get one of those computer viruses."

10) Cryptogenic - like the odd Cryptogenic Organizing Pneumonia Mimicking Hydatid Disease. Cryptogenic means hidden cause. "This is so mysterious, we have hardly a clue."

11) Acronymous - diseases like AIDS, SARS, and SIDS may be so obtuse that they need long names, like COPMHD above. Acronyms can make diseases more manageable at least for charting purposes.

12) Asymptomatic - as in asymptomatic hepatitis in which the "disease" shows only on tests. "You look well and seem well, but one of those routine tests we did came up with an abnormal result. Because of which we will most definitely have to do further ones."

13) Spontaneous - as in conditions which arise without warning or apparent cause. Medics can add "Spontaneous" in front of the rest of the label.

14) Idiosyncratic - as in one of a kind. "We have never seen anything quite like this before. We are having a time deciding why it happened to you. And we may need more time."

15) Allergic - as in reaction. "Your body is reacting abnormally. This is surely due to foreign substances that don't bother most people. We

don't know why this situation has developed at this time. But, we sure can do some testing and maybe some treatment against that substance which has begun to disturb you for who knows what reason."

16) Autoimmune - refers to diseases or syndromes in which the body seems to attack its own cells and tissues. There are literally dozens of these conditions which medicine minutely studies and describes demonstrating that "We Still Don't Know."

17) Latinized - as in encephalitis. Rather than say brain fever, used a century ago, the Latin term sounds more professional and impressive.

18) -itis - referring to the suffix as in encephalitis. Just tack -itis onto any Latin name for a body part and you have a disease. But typically of unknown cause. -itis refers to inflammation.

19) -osis - like halitosis or keratosis. -osis just means an abnormal condition, disease or accentuation of a body part or process. It sounds more professional than bad breath or thickening of skin.

20) -pathy - like cardiomyopathy. Put -pathy together at the end of a word to name a condition which is usually scary, persistent and relatively untreatable. -pathy is a Latin term meaning disease.

21) Rheumatic or rheumatoid - as in fever or arthritis. These names suggest that the whole body is involved, thus a systemic disease. Source usually undetermined.

22) Descriptive - as in Sudden Infant Death Syndrome (SIDS). Many diagnoses are just mere descriptions of what the physician understands from symptoms and tests, or thinks s/he understands.

23) Congenital - as in birth defect. "He was born with it. We don't know why. There is nothing we can do about it. It is congenital, maybe in the genes. He will have to learn to live with it."

24) Familial - as in Familial Hypercholesterolemia. "It runs in the family and is hereditary. Let's blame it on the ancestors!"

25) Hereditary - as in hemophilia. "We have found the genes which sometimes, but not always causes this problem. We are doing further studies to expand understanding and hopefully treatment."

26) Genetic - as in definitely familial-hereditary and identifiable by a genetic marker. "We think we understand the cause. We have found a gene which may be important. But we still can't do much about your

problem. Keep checking with us." Genes and DNA are in these days. But, don't they really lead us to dead ends? What creates genes, genetic material, DNA?

27) Incurable - as in many of the above mentioned diseases. But, what makes a disease incurable? And who says it so?

28) Terminal - incurable diseases often become terminal. But then, everything is terminal. Even the earth and sun and stars come and go. Things are temporary. What continues? Another good question.

Let's "examine" the disease known as Ankylosing Spondylitis as an example which touches on many of those listed above. This was the incurable (27) disease with which Norman Cousins (see Hospital Time) was diagnosed.

Ankylosing spondylitis is a combination of ankylosis (19) and spondylitis (18). Vertebral (spondylos) and pelvic joints become inflamed (-itis) and may stiffen (-osis) to the point of fusion.

AS is also called Marie-Strumpell (7) disease or Bekhterev's (7) disease or Bekhterev's syndrome (6). Ankylosing spondylitis is a spondyloarthropathy (20), meaning it affects the vertebral joints.

AS is a rheumatic (21) disease. It affects the whole body. In other words, AS is a type of rheumatoid arthritis (18). AS and RA are both typically incurable (27) and sometimes terminal (28).

A number of genes (26) are implicated but not proven to cause the disease, bringing cure or relief no closer.

There have been longstanding claims that antigens (15) of the Klebsiella bacteria are involved in causation. But, not proven.

One positive thing we can say about Ankylosing Spondylitis is that Norman Cousins was "healed" of it largely through his own intuitions, efforts, will to live and grow.

Interestingly, Norman Cousins gave great praise to his physician in his recovery. "If I had to guess, I would say that the principal contribution made by my doctor to the taming, and possibly the conquest, of my illness was that he encouraged me to believe I was a respected partner with him in the total undertaking. He fully engaged my subjective energies. He may not have been able to define or diagnose the process through which self-confidence (wild hunches securely believed) was somehow picked up by the body's immunologic mechanisms and translated into anti-morbid effects. But he was acting, I believe, in the best tradition of medicine in recognizing that he had to reach out in my case beyond the usual verifiable modalities. In so doing, he was faithful to the first dictum in medical education: *primum non nocere*. He knew that what I wanted to do might not help, but it probably would do little harm. Certainly, the threatened harm being risked was less if anything, than the heroic medication so routinely administered in extreme cases of this kind." (*Anatomy of an Illness*)

There is one very common kind of disease of which WE DO KNOW the cause. But, it is little discussed and little addressed. Certainly not to the degree of many of the labels just listed. It is called iatrogenic illness. Using Greek terms, iatro meaning healer and genic referring to causation, we can quickly get to the bottom of a host of medical problems which result from physician tests, prescriptions, operations, treatments, hospitalization and the like.

If medics were less obsessed with identification and intervention, they would need a lot less disease labels mentioned above and have to deal with far fewer iatrogenic disorders.

A Frugal Physician is not a slave to labels, names and diagnoses. Like any or all of the above. S/he is concerned with people. S/he understands that illness is a complicated mix of physical, mental-emotional, spiritual, social energies playing upon a person at any one time. An FP won't spend a lot of your time and money on tests nor in diagnosis unless you deem it necessary.

Name Your Poison

First, do no harm (*primum non nocere*), is surely the Father of Medicine's most important recommendation. A Frugal Physician recognizes this and tries to uphold this teaching simply because s/he knows that there is far greater wisdom beyond him/herself in creation, in life, and often in disease. Even with the wonders of modern times, it is hard to outwit nature. So, it is often best to "back off and let time and nature attend to things."

Unfortunately, the commercial way of the world which pervades medicine requires it to have something in stock for every occasion. Medicine has become like a grocery story with treatments for practically everything. Physicians could well put an advertisement on their literature: "We treat everything."

Medicine has "expropriated health," as Ivan Illich says, and expanded its domain into far reaches of modern life. Of course, much of this expropriation surrounds disease. But, it goes on to penetrate and invade much of human affairs just like government has done.

Medics treat almost everything. The exceptions are most often those that are thought to be "mental" in origin. If symptoms don't jive with physical signs and tests or the "patient is a bit light in the head," then his/her problem is unreal or psychological in nature. A "shrink" or "head specialist" is needed.

Appropriate referral is then in order and the Regular Physician can go back to his Regular Patients. The doctor no doubt has enough of those to work with.

But then, how is one - any one - any physician - to know what is a valid complaint. What is real?

Doesn't that depend on who is asking and who is answering? Once a physician has become a patient, s/he may begin to think differently on the subject.

Regardless, a person might want to know what constitutes a Real Disease after having gone through the long list of Diseases in Name

Only. Let me not give the impression that those patients who are given any of the diagnoses listed in the previous chapter have no valid complaints. Far from it.

The author's experience suggest that malingerers are quite uncommon in clinics and hospitals. Patients rarely "make up diseases." We certainly do have hypochondriacs in our midst. In past eras, they were called hysterics or neurasthenics. Now, they are usually called neurotics. It is more gently and politically correct to call them "prone to anxiety" or "easily depressed" and to prescribe Valium or Paxil.

All of these patients have REAL problems. However, Regular Physicians are quite often not astute enough and the system not flexible enough to tune into the true sources of their problems. They keep searching for causes in the material bodies of their patients. "Well, all those tests we did came up absolutely normal." Can you guess what that means, when the tests are normal but the patient continues to have problems and to complain? Either more tests or a mental health evaluation.

Doctors and patients continue to expend vast amounts of energy and money chasing after those elusive and illusory diagnoses. They empower sets of symptoms by giving them scary names which tend to magnify fears all around.

In truth, real medicine and true healing "ignores disease as-an-object" and also "gives freedom, power and happiness." (Richard Grossinger) The latter is a tall order to be sure, but one that a Frugal Physician considers generally true and widely applicable.

The point is that patients have vast ranges of experiences and symptoms which physicians awkwardly pigeonhole, name, and treat. This is a major concept which physicians and public need to understand. Natural life is neither as simple as we try to make it nor as complicated as it becomes in the course of chasing illusive diagnoses.

Most illnesses do not have single causes and straightforward treatments. Most develop over time and become prominent at strategic passages in life. They can be at best met only partially from the medical angle. Life itself is a healing process. And disease is part of that process. Paradoxical as it may seem.

But, the medical profession has long proclaimed practically all symptoms of discomfort the enemy and gone into battle with ever stronger and bigger weapons - to fight the good fight.

We fight disease like we fight wars, too often with overwhelming force which may be more damaging to the patient than his original problem. Consider for a moment the tools of medicine used over the ages, many of which seem to have brought numerous ill ones through death's door prematurely.

How often does medicine conjure diseases to treat rather than deal with the reality of the patient's life and situation? How often does the Emperor of the Kingdom of Disease have no clothes?

Physicians and patients alike give power and honor to Disease and all who serve the Ruler. This is totally understandable for patients who react to pain and anxiety and ignorance. "This looks bad, feels worse and could be very serious."

Physicians so often add to patient problems, by naming and labeling. If you have a "real disease," your physician will surely come up with a "real name" for it. Patients can be just as adamant in the naming and empowering process.

When you claim or accept a disease label, you have got it for as long as you want. Maybe the rest of your life. There are so many examples. Real or not, when a diagnostic label is put on a disease or symptom complex, it is likely to stick. Here are a few:

- I remember seeing a car parked at one of the clinics where I worked years ago. The personalized license plate read LUPUS. "Ouch!" I told myself, "Now, there is someone who is committed to her disease."

I got the story from a third party that the owner of the car was a patient with an obvious ailment (lupus erythematosus) and also president of the local society of the same name. Nothing like promoting your disease!

I am sure she meant well, trying to promote her cause and advertise it on the front and back of her auto. But with that kind of thinking, she was certain to carry the label as well as the symptoms of lupus until her dying day.

Whatever forces brought LUPUS into that woman's life were reinforced by her absorbing the label, having it on an office door and letterhead, wearing it on her name badge, and putting it on her personal license plate. How could anyone ever let go, give up an identity like that? Good for her or not, the person surely had become identified with her disease.

• Labeling is a bottom line feature of the Anonymous programs. AA members always introduce whatever they have to say in meetings with words like, "I'm Joe and I'm an alcoholic."

For many members that is a powerful statement. It generally suggests an individual who has stopped to take a good look at himself - at least for a time, admitted defeat, and "turned his life over to a Higher Power."

That is surely a huge step. But, it is also only a step. That label ALCOHOLIC, held too tightly, can become so potent that it keeps the individual an alcoholic and prevents growth to another level. How about saying something like, "Hi, I'm Joe. I am no longer an alcoholic. I am a healthy human being." Let Joe identify himself with a deeper, truer part of his being. He may be better off dispensing altogether with the word ALCOHOLIC and allowing it to fade totally into the past.

There are stories about the On-and-On Anonymous Programs because there are so many different ones out there. Some of these people become addicted to 12-Step Programs. Again, that is a step up from the original addiction. But, aren't there more steps?

• This naming practice goes around and around in words and the intimations which surround them. "I'm a diabetic and always will be." "I have arthritis. I own the disease and it owns me." "I have cancer. It will probably kill me or I will die trying to get rid of it."

The power of naming can be recognized in many ways and places. Just as much if not more so in modern times because we need names and labels to put on our paperwork, get insurance coverage, and justify sick leave.

The old adage of "Sticks and stones may break my bones, but words will never hurt me," is obviously untrue. Words and titles can empower as well as disable.

A whole book could be written on the topic of "What's in a Name." Name calling certainly has its effects. Immediate and long term. For good or ill. Think about your own birth name, how you have carried it and how it suits you or not. Do you identify with the name you were given? What if you were a Boy Named Sue?

Here is a secondhand story. One I heard while I was on the road leading workshops in the 90s. I sat in on a weekly class prior to my own program at the site of my upcoming venue and heard this anecdote which the leader told on herself. Sylvia recounted how she had started the ball rolling with what she had thought was a harmless joke. But, she repeated her joke many times to friends and, in particular, to family members who were followers of evangelist Oral Roberts. Her intention was to get a rise out of her kin. But, it sure backfired.

With animation and theatrics, Sylvia told that Oral had died and gone to heaven. He was immediately greeted by Saint Peter. When Saint Peter discovered who his new guest was, he was elated and overjoyed. "THE Oral Roberts? Oh, my. Are we glad to see you. We have been looking forward to your joining us."

Saint Peter eventually got the word through Jesus on up the line and Oral was invited to stand before the Almighty. Roberts was thrilled and humbled at the same time. Soon, he was brought into the Almighty's Presence. After just a few pleasantries and bows, GOD stared beseechingly at the newcomer for a moment. "Oral. Oral. I need your help. Yes, I do."

"Anything I can do, My LORD. Please say it and it will be as good as done."

GOD pointed to HIS shoulder and said, "Oral. Oral, I have a pain right here."

The story was funny. It probably didn't go over well with her family members. But, it boomeranged on Sylvia. In the midst of her repeated tale telling, Sylvia developed a frozen shoulder - in that same shoulder to which she pointed time and again. She eventually took herself to see an orthopedist for help. (Roberts wasn't available.) It was quite a learning opportunity and Sylvia was repentant, at least for the moment.

Interestingly, Sylvia never called her shoulder names. But, she made it clear that it was not okay.

People - who often become patients - are apt to give names to parts of their bodies which are not working up to their standards. I have tried to influence people who say, "This is my bad shoulder." Or, "That old bum leg of mine."

The person might do better saying, "This shoulder doesn't work like the other one, or the way it used to . . ."

I can assure him or her that that part of his or her anatomy is still performing quite amazingly (from various perspectives), doing much of its intended work, and continues very largely healthy. It just isn't functioning as usual.

- Disabled is another label becoming more and more common. It is not politically correct to be Crippled, but it is okay to be Disabled. Actually, it is a bonanza for many because a government check and release from labor often goes with it. More and more people are taking the Disabled route to early retirement. This seems to be an interesting but often sad state of affairs.

Early in my teaching days, I interviewed a middle-aged woman named Flo whose life had been difficult. Still, she had her religious beliefs, personal studies, and varied interests.

While attending the classes I taught, Flo gave a number of hints like, "I have been told that I have some healing abilities. I just haven't been able to develop them." At the same time, Flo had some unnamed ailment which might get her a "Disability." She had had enough of menial jobs and was hoping to give them up and settle in with a Disability check.

There seemed to be a bit of a conflict. So at one point in private, I had to ask her, "Which is most important to you? Developing your healing abilities or getting a disability check."

"I am embarrassed to say that the check is." A tough choice. But, Flo would be labeled as Disabled rather than Healer. Consider the implications.

- Another label which the medical - or psychiatry - profession seems intent on spreading around is already very common: DEPRESSION. We now have National Depression Week and the media regularly tries to get people to take a quick Depression Quiz so early treatment can be started.

For a time, I worked with a hypnotist named Sam Meranto in Phoenix, Arizona. He was more of a businessman than a therapist, but Sam also had charisma which helped in his work, attracted clients, and gave them hopes for the future.

On one particular day, I was interviewing a client. As the hypnotist walked in on our conversation, I was saying, "You seem a bit depressed today."

Sam got animated and joined the talk, "No, no! You should never say, 'You look depressed.' Instead say something like, 'You look good, but you could look better.'" The thought had merit and begged further consideration.

By the way, one of the best things that Mr. Sam Meranto did was to help people discard labels which they had attracted and accepted over the years.

- Sam told a story which concerns a common, simple every day label. From his factory working days back East, he recalled a time when he wanted to prove a point.

He got three friends to "gang up" on another named Mack. First thing in the morning, one of the three went up to talk to Mack. As soon as he turned around, the man said, "Oh my God, Mack. You don't look so good. You must be sick. Are you okay?" Mack denied any illness.

An hour later, another of the group encountered Mack and said, "Hey, how are ya doin'? You look a little green around the gills. Are you all right?" Mack said he was fine.

A third and then a fourth confederate told Joe much the same.

Before noon, Mack checked out and went home SICK.

Sick is another label which has many ways of insinuating itself into our lives. Meranto's rejoinder to his story was that," Whenever anything negative is spoken to you or at you, you should neutralize it with opposite words at least three times."

- Mr. Meranto was keenly against such labels as ... "You're fat." "He's a basket case." "She's a druggie." "The old gomer." More and more labels which bear neutralization or dismissal.

These names remind me of my maiden aunt Em, who had a few problems. Mostly of her own making, like the rest of us. She had lived close to 60 years by herself and collected peculiarities which were not always noticeable because of her singular life.

Auntie Em kept a little cartoon glued to her bathroom medicine cabinet mirror. Every time she stared into the mirror, the card read back to her, "You've got a very unusual kind of face. It's the stupid kind."

Labels are surely here to stay for a long time to come. But if we insist on labels, maybe we can come up with some better ones.

- If you want to scare someone, tell him he has cancer or will get it. Put the hex on him. There aren't many bigger bogeys out there than cancer. Cancer has so many victims.

Cancer patients are VICTIMS, are they not? We hear it so often and people with that diagnosis generally act accordingly.

Victims are dis-empowered, terrorized in a variety of ways - physical, psychological and otherwise. Too often they are made or become pushovers to their disease.

Cancer is most distressing, for sure, because it very often has the potential to be TERMINAL. Another label. How many more labels do we need?

Disease Rights

Terminal, incurable and hopeless labels seem to go together. But, aren't they all in the eyes of the beholder - physician or patient? Here is a story that puts a striking twist on the whole issue.

Years ago when I first joined the staff of the A.R.E. (Association for Research and Enlightenment) Clinic in Phoenix, Arizona, I was given the task of answering phone messages and letters from people new to our organization. The writers and callers often had unusual inquiries for our equally unusual clinic.

A memorable letter came in from a Mr. Graves from North Carolina. He immediately started by complaining about our parent organization back in Virginia. Nonetheless, he continued on in his letter telling about his two incurable diseases and asking for recommendations via the mail.

Mr. Graves had been to Duke Medical Center, consulted all manner of specialists and even seen faith healers and other non-traditional health workers. Nothing helped and he continued to suffer with his TWO "incurable illnesses."

I remember reading his note and thinking, "This fellow has a lot of gall to be complaining on the one hand about our organization and on the other asking for help - for free and long distance - for his TWO "incurable diseases."

Still, I sat down and wrote him a full letter starting like this:

"Dear Mr. Graves, Thank you for your letter and comments. I can tell by the way you write that you are a frank and direct person. Let me be equally direct with you. Mr. Cayce (the founder of A.R.E.) is remembered for saying that 'there are no incurable illnesses, only incurable people.' I would like for you to consider that idea and see if you can work at becoming a curable person. Then, you will be much better able to deal with your health concerns. . . ."

I sent the letter out and was surprised to get a response in what seemed to be record speed for cross country mail delivery. Mr. Graves thanked me for my note. He quickly added. "I made a mistake. I don't have two incurable illnesses. I have three."

Not TWO "incurable" diseases, but THREE. Wow! How would you respond to that? Honestly, I don't remember how I did. But obviously, Mr. Graves hadn't gotten the message. He was likely to stay in the "incurable person" category.

The idea of an incurable disease seems to be simple and straightforward at first glance. But on further consideration, "incurable" falls into the same category as "disease" itself.

"Incurable" like "disease" itself does not stand direct scrutiny. Cross examination tears them both apart. Incurable even more so than disease.

We have already seen many holes poked into the idea of Disease. More are coming. DISEASE is bleeding from many sites. There is one gaping wound in the side of Incurable. It is simply this: If a single solitary human has ever been "cured" of a disease, syndrome, ailment, or condition, then it is simply not "incurable."

From that view, there are for all practical purposes no incurable medical conditions. Even death is subject to "cure." Dead folks sit up in their coffins. Infants revive after their breathing has stopped. People throughout history have risen from the dead. Yogis have been interred and entombed for weeks at a time - certainly dead to world, and later drawn back to the realm of the living.

On a broad basis, the term "incurable" is clearly inaccurate. At least as far as disease is considered.

The other side of Mr. Grave's story is about the curability of people and really bears much more thought and contemplation. It begs the question, "What makes one person curable and the other not? The one to live and the other die from a similar scenario."

Mr. Graves was/is not alone in his futile search for real help with his major medical problems. With the cooperation of Medical Authorities, he surely found lots of company because of all the "incurable diseases" around.

Graves most certainly had very real problems, but they weren't curable in the context of the present medical model. Nor were they understandable. A Frugal Physician works to see through the myth of DISEASE and help people become curable. That, however, is much easier imagined than done.

It was not long after my correspondence with Mr. Graves, that I encountered another extraordinary patient face to face. Unique was an apt adjective for the A.R.E. Clinic as well as many of its patients who were drawn from the around the country to its one-week and two-week-long healing programs. The patients in the programs stayed in the Oak House which was located a few blocks from the clinic. They exercised, prayed and meditated, and ate meals together. A physician was in attendance at every meal during which time people recited their night time dreams, related their life stories, and recalled trials and triumphs.

The program was quite innovative and attracted a broad spectrum of people including a woman named Patsy. While Patsy didn't appear to have a "Real Disease," her predicament was totally real and engaging. Sadly, we medics were not sharp enough to come up with a way to help her.

One Friday afternoon at the clinic, I consulted with this 30-year-old woman from Georgia who wanted to participate in the next healing program. She had been "recruited" at a conference in San Diego. Still, I was warned ahead of time that Patsy was not a typical patient and might not quite "fit in." I was to determine her suitability before the program day began.

As soon as I met the tall, blondish, brusque woman, Patsy handed me a list of ten (10) diseases which she believed she had and hoped we could help her with. Her main concern however was CANCER which was at the top of her list. Patsy's understanding of her cancer was strangely limited. She didn't know what kind of cancer she had or where it originated. She just knew, "I've got cancer and the Army caused it, but they won't help me." (She had been on active military duty working in a hospital some years previously.)

We completed an "exploratory" consultation with plans for a return visit on Monday. In the meantime, I was able to contact the woman's psychiatrist who had been treating her for many months. He told me that Patsy had never been diagnosed with cancer and was really in quite good physical health. It was clearly her mind that was the problem.

This information was coupled with news that Patsy had had a panic attack when she was driven to her motel after the clinic visit. (Blinds on the car windows meant to keep the Arizona sun out made Patsy think she was in jail). It was quite clear that the young Georgian would definitely not "fit in" the planned healing program. I was, however, a bit anxious about telling Patsy that we couldn't admit her to the program. I asked another young physician, Joe, to join me while I told Patsy the not-so-good news.

I said something like, "We feel that the program is not suited for you. We will be happy to see you on an individual basis to help you with your problems." This pronouncement disturbed her greatly and she struggled to get us to change the plan.

Eventually, the conversation got around to "cancer" and we had to tell her that we had no evidence that she had such a disease. This admission incensed her even more.

After we parted, Joe and I went into the doctors' den and pondered on what had just happened. I felt like we had had no choice in our decision. Out of the blue, Joe said, "You know, Bob, we might have missed it. There was another possibility. We could have treated her for cancer. We should have been able to manage a cure since she doesn't have the disease to begin with. We should have been able to come up with some treatment plan and convince her into making it work."

For a moment, he had me, "Wow! You might be onto something. Maybe we blew it." Then, I recalled that list she had handed me on Friday afternoon.

I pulled Patsy's list from her chart and reminded him. I said, "Interesting thought, Joe. But, her problems go beyond cancer. You know, this list has nine other diseases on it. If we 'cured her cancer,' that would be just the beginning. She might even have more lists stashed away."

Patsy was clearly caught in a powerful aura of disease. She and Disease had "A thing going on." What was she drawing to her?

Mr. Graves and Patsy had more than a few things in common. Both had so-called incurable illnesses with typical implications. Both seemed to have latched onto their diseases - real or unreal, physical or mental - with powerful grips. However their medical problems had developed, Graves and Patsy were determined to hang onto them - although they surely would have said otherwise.

While most patients believe they want to be rid of their ailments, many unconsciously express their Right to Disease. Paradoxically, this is pretty much in accord with the way medicine often works. Physicians "intend" to make sick people well, the injured able. But, the system of practice often promotes the opposite. The more we focus on disease, the more it clings for life.

A Frugal Physician recognizes that patients and their diseases pair up in a meaningful fashion. Just as physicians and patients do. Regular Physicians stand unconsciously with disease in so many ways. A Frugal Physician has his/her work cut out to bring forth a workable paradigm of health and healing.

Purple Pills and Magic Bullets

Regular Physicians seem to have "A pill for every ill." If all those pills really did what they were supposed to do and without side effects, the human race would have much less discomfort and life would be a whole lot easier on us.

Rational, thinking people realize life is not that simple. All is not as it appears or is advertised. What is intended for our good is not always so. Obviously, medications quite often do not live up to the specifications, promotions and advertisements behind them.

Like government fixes, medics and their system are supposed to help. They often REALLY want to help. But, methods and practice rarely stack up with intentions.

Help is clearly not always helpful. There are two sides to every coin. Sometimes, it seems like more than two. In the case of medical practice, it seems that the coin is more like a multi-hedron. Like a many-sided die which tends to be easily pushed onto a different side after it is first thrown.

Interestingly in the present era, the word medicine has at least a dual meaning. The obvious refers to the profession which deals with treatment of disease. The second involves potions and pills most generally taken by mouth in those treatments. "Take your medicine whether it's good for you or not."

Medicine and medication are practically synonymous in recent generations. Pills are the preferred and sometimes, it seems, the only acceptable method in treating modern ailments. No wonder we are a pill popping society!

In his professional days, one of the author's major discomforts with medical practice was its one-dimensional nature. Its singular focus on the body which goes along with material - chemical and mechanical - treatments, most often medicines.

As a young physician, his choices (being in training and watched over by the all-powerful guild) were often between prescribing penicillin or ampicillin. Or, nothing at all. The latter was generally a better choice. But often, neither appreciated nor understood by patients and other physicians.

"In the Church of Modern Medicine, the doctor who treats without drugs is regarded as a heretic because he or she appears to have rejected the sacrament of medication. Non-drug healers are regarded as belonging to a different religious system and are thought of as quacks, nuts or faddists." (Robert Mendelsohn)

My sense was that I had worked my way into a very narrow, limited, and non-creative if not often destructive profession. Most of our treatments - and especially our MEDICINES - were and are antagonistic to body functions. Antagonists work against the body and its usual actions.

When a person takes a medication, s/he generally has two if not three problems to deal with. His/her original complaint plus the effects and side effects of the medication. If one problem isn't enough, you as patient will have at least two when you depart your doctor's office.

Here is another quick list for your consideration. This one is of common types of drugs.

anti-allergics	anti-tussives	anti-depressants
anti-cholinergics	anti-cholinesterases	anti-biotics
anti-diarrheals	anti-adrenergics	anti-spasmodics

ant-helminthics	anti-hypertensives	anti-inflammatories
anti-arrhythmics	anti-infectives	anti-cholesteremics
anti-convulsants	anti-pyretics	anti-diabetics
anti-arthritics	anti-asthmatics	anti-septics

This list really could go on and on. Interestingly, a list of "pro" type medications, ones intended to support and enhance body functions, would be on the order of one tenth the length of "anti" medicines. Such medications are also newer, generally less known, and infrequently prescribed.

Drugs and the chemicals from which they are made very often do not accomplish the task they are meant to take on. Most simply because all bodies do not react the same to medications. And with every action, there is a reaction. The suppression of one symptom is likely to create another - sooner or later.

Medications are developed under laboratory conditions. Human beings live under human conditions. No wonder the real life experience of taking drugs often does not follow the patterns set in drug trials and testing.

Physicians and their patients don't really relate to the years involved in drug testing. They are often looking for quick fixes and ready remedies. "The faster the better, so I can get back to regular life." This aspect of modern life often adds to problems, as symbolized in the television commercial which shows Vanquish taking care of a headache in a hurry. Is that how real life works?

Certain age groups are well known to experience more troubles with medications. Particularly the older population because they consume so many.

SPECIAL POEM FOR SENIOR CITIZENS
(Anonymous)

A row of bottles on my shelf
Caused me to analyze myself.
One yellow pill I have to pop

> Goes to my heart so it won't stop.
> A little white one that I take
> Goes to my hands so they won't shake.
>
> The blue ones that I use a lot
> Tell me I'm happy when I'm not.
> The purple pill goes to my brain
> and tells me that I have no pain.
> The capsules tell me not to wheeze
> Or cough or choke or even sneeze.
> The red ones, smallest of them all
> Go to my blood so I won't fall.
> The orange ones, very big and bright
> Prevent my leg cramps in the night.
> Such an array of brilliant pills
> Helping to cure all kinds of ills.
> But what I'd really like to know...........
> Is what tells each one where to go!

Yeah, where DO they go? If medical science is so advanced, why do almost all medications circulate through the whole bloodstream and affect the whole system when most of the time the patient is complaining about an ache here, an upset there, or a discomfort somewhere else? Not all over.

The numbers of medications which some older people take can be staggering and downright scary. Especially when those patients see more than one physician.

Sometimes, the best remedy for an elder person is to take him or her off all medication and start all over. A daunting process in itself, discontinuing medication is often the last thing which a Regular Physician will try. Where medications are considered, physicians are uniformly more comfortable with addition rather than subtraction. Besides, they started the process. Reversing course may not look so good to patient and family members.

Discontinuing medication can really frighten the patient and his/her family as they wonder about the consequences of drug withdrawal. "Were those drugs ever useful or necessary? How much did we spend on them?"

The physician has qualms and concerns because s/he has no way of predicting what will happen when the medication is discontinued. Even more so when several are stopped or tapered at the same time. That said, a regimen of tapering medications is a sure way to keep the patient visiting the clinic regularly.

Medics definitely don't like to take people off their pills. They feel safer with "the usual regimen," whether helpful to the patient or not. Prescribing is relatively simple. Stopping a medication has a host of uncomfortable implications.

Polypharmacy (sounds like a new drugstore chain, doesn't it?) refers to patients who take multiple medications. This is a whole arena of modern medicine which has become an area of common concern. It persists and continues to grow as does the lucrative pharmaceutical industry.

The major problem with polypharmacy is simple. Physicians and pharmacists are often uncertain about the risks and effects of a single medication in one patient's body. When more chemicals are added to the human body which is already under stress, the interactions of the drugs are often totally unknown. All the while, the body is called upon to metabolize a host of waste products beyond the usual.

But, the desire for remedies in pill form persist. "Pills are popular" with patients and practitioners.

The height of pill-pushing seems to have arrived with Nexium, the Purple Pill, a preparation for heartburn made by Astra Zeneca. Pharmaceutical companies have used marketing gimmicks to get the public's attention - as well as the physician's - for decades. But, the Purple Pill deserves a prize. It does have a ring to it, but the ploy is clearly the height of hype.

Pharmaceutical companies have been literally sugar-coating their medications for a long time. Along the way, they have spent huge monies in coming up with exotic names. Have you ever noticed how many drugs have Xs and Ys and Zs in their names? How does a catchy name for a pill make it more useful or effective?

The Purple Pill obviously and blatantly puts cosmetics above substance. "Try our Purple Pills. They will not only help your stomach but also go well in your medicine chest or pill box and even serve as table ornaments. Take Purple Pills with you anywhere. They will brighten up most any decor."

I am reminded of an incident some years ago with an old friend, since passed away. Dan Henning was a college professor nearing retirement who had overcome his alcohol addiction in a relatively novel way. He was warm, funny, sincere and generous, but also tall, gangly, awkward, and needy. Henning was quite affectionately and accurately known as Big Foot.

Dan came to every class I taught. I might have been flattered, but I knew that he went to many, many self-help classes. He attended 12-step programs, supported all kinds of therapists, and took every workshop that came down the pike.

I visited him at his home a few times and found all kinds of health oriented books piled here and there. He had many bottles of vitamins visible in the kitchen and bathroom.

Dan subscribed to the idea that, "If one is good, two is better." This became clear as I noticed he had TWO tape players running non-stop with TWO different subliminal tapes buzzing away. Curiously, Dan was hard of hearing and wore aides in both ears.

Dr. Dan often appeared at class sessions with something to share. I will never forget the evening he came to a session and proudly displayed a tiny bottle which contained "healing oil which was expressed from the bones of a dead nun."

That stopped me in my tracks to the point that I had to remark, "Wow! Dan, you've tried so many of these things, been to so many workshops and classes and therapists. You ought to write a book about your experiences."

Henning chuckled and responded, "Yeah, Bob, I think you're right. I might do that. I would call it 'Gullible's Travels.'"

Dan and you and I are more alike than we might admit. We just choose different treatments to believe in. Dan believed in alternative approaches. Practically all of them. Oh, he also went to Regular Physicians. Most of them were surgeons.

When thinking of drugs and pharmaceuticals, there are so many issues of which the Frugal Physician and his patients should be aware. Here is another partial list:

• Iatrogenic (physician-caused) disease is more common than even researchers want to know. The use of prescription drugs is largely overdone and the system doesn't keep up with the plethora of pills in patient hands. Much to the detriment of the patient population. Ten to 20 percent of hospital admissions are known to be due to adverse drug reactions (ADRs) and other ill effects of medication.

Recurring research studies repeatedly show that testing, medication, surgery and hospitalization are overused and dangerous to patient health. Alas! That information does not filter well into medical training or practice. It rarely gets into patients' hands.

• Warnings are commonly made about pregnant women taking medications. Those warnings may be useful for that population.

But, they seem to make the rest of us second class citizens with regard to drug safety. If drugs can be harmful to the pregnant and the newborn, they also may be harmful for the rest of us. Shouldn't we all be protected against the dangers of drug prescription?

• On the other hand for some patients (remember everyone is different), medication does not build up in the system. Instead, it is metabolized so quickly and efficiently by the body that it is likely to have little or no effect.

Or, the body may simply get used to the drug's presence. Sometimes, requiring increased dosage. Some people can become habituated to their meds like drinkers do with alcohol. Regular intake may have no effect at all on the body. The patient may just get accustomed to the situation thinking, "I must be getting some benefit out of this prescription."

That medication you have been taking and paying well for may have absolutely no effect on your body. Your feeling or behaving better may be caused by a dozen different things which have nothing to do with medication.

• Trial and Error. It is typical for the Regular Physician to say, "Let's give this new medicine a TRY for a couple weeks. If it doesn't work, we will TRY something else later." Haven't you heard that a few times? Your physician is just practicing, but maybe you should expect more savvy in his methods and practice.

• While the FDA mandates primarily for safety when passing on new drugs, efficacy is less important. Even then, how many drugs show up years later to be implicated in one serious problem or another?
Some human beings take the same medication for years and it may take years for ill effects to appear. How many drug makers value the consumers' health and welfare to test their medications with humans, day-to-day, in real life situations for many years prior to pumping their new med into the market?

• The Food and Drug Administration doesn't make pharmaceutical companies prove that their new medicine is effective - that they really do what they are prescribed for. Proof of safety is hard enough. Proof of REAL efficacy is not required to get medication on the pharmacist's counter and in your doctor's office.
The law requires "substantial evidence of effectiveness" to okay a new drug. At the same time, it says "relative efficacy" is sufficient and the FDA may not disapprove a drug on the grounds that a more effective option is available. The question of "relative efficacy" is a big one which has not been well answered for over 40 years. How can you or anyone really know that the new prescription just filled is effective or even safe?

• We clearly live in a pill culture. Trillions of pills are prescribed every year costing around $300 billion in the USA alone. That figure does not include the over-the-counter market which has grown substantially in recent years. Again, there is a pill for every ill. How does that way of living effect young people who are bombarded with pill mentality from early on?

What kind of a message do we send to young people? "You need to take Ritalin, but you're too young to drink alcohol." "I am going to the pharmacy to refill your psychotropic drugs. I don't want to smell cigarette smoke when I get back home." "That weed you've been smoking is illegal and going to get you in trouble. It will lead to heroin." Or, maybe back to Ritalin.

- Our friend, Dr. Hippocrates told us long ago to "Let food be your medicine and medicine be your food." Why do we persist in looking for answers in little colored pills if answers may be found in our foods? (Actually, medics are trying harder to find other routes besides pills to make things easier for patients. Like patches and long-term injections, etc.)

Unfortunately, nutrition was little discussed when I went to medical school. I remember it being announced at some point that we had been given twenty (20) hours of nutrition during our thousands of hours of classroom basic science courses.

But, I sure didn't recall even an approximation thereof. In two areas, we got bits and pieces of nutrition. Pathology: we were given some information on diseases which appear in extremes of malnutrition, such as scurvy, beriberi, pellagra, etc. Surgery: Dr. Stanley Dudrick was a leader in parenteral nutrition at our medical school at the time. He was a surgeon and was working on ways for surgical patients to be "fed" through the intravenous route during prolonged periods in which they could not take food by mouth.

It was laudable work, but little applicable to most medical practice then or now. Fortunately, few people will have to live for long periods only on such nutritional elements.

Pharmaceuticals far, far outweigh foods in medical training and practice. Trying to compare their importance to modern medicine seems ludicrous. Nutrition presently has no place in medicine for all practical purposes.

I am reminded of when my mother was dying of breast cancer. She wouldn't dare take an aspirin or a vitamin without consulting her physician. My older brother wanted her to take some of his Herbalife products, but she wouldn't hear of it. "The doctor would have to say it's okay."

One day, medical orthodoxy suggests that vitamins and nutritional preparations are innocuous or useless. "Don't waste your money." On the next, they suggest that they might be dangerous and interfere with medications they prescribe.

- It is IMPORTANT to note that practically every medication in the books - or one like it - is naturally produced in the human body. If it doesn't, it surely has the innate capability. The human form is constantly reproducing itself, constructing and re-constructing. Like other living creatures, the human organism miraculously takes a few simple building blocks and transforms - probably transmutes others to keep its structure intact and its functioning uniform over decades of use.

If man can make a drug in the laboratory, the human body most certainly makes something like it already. Science obviously should put more of a focus on what the body does and does rightly in the vast majority of its lifespan.

- If a human body can make a small amount of a substance, why not a "normal" amount. At the first hint of hypothyroidism, physicians place the patient on a synthetic thyroid hormone (often for years or a lifetime). The synthetic is a takeoff on the original.

If the body is already making some of the hormone (which is quite likely even after surgery or irradiation), why don't physicians help, teach, stimulate the body to produce more adequately, functionally, and normally?

Drugs and medications have a place in the modern world - albeit a much smaller one in a more perfect world. But, the plethora of drugs for this, that and practically every purpose seems wildly out of hand, wasteful and unnecessary. And then, potentially dangerous and harmful as well.

- Magic bullets. A whole book could be written about these medications. Actually, many have already been so written on antibiotics and steroids. But, few if any from a critical point of view.

  First, physicians use these drugs with an attitude something akin to "We'll knock 'em dead and clear 'em out." It is never that simple. Both kinds of chemicals are destructive and antagonistic drugs, anti-biotics and anti-inflammatories being their main usage. If antibiotics kill bacteria, they certainly can and do have negative effects upon other cells which they contact as they circulate through the whole body. If they don't have any effect on normal tissues, then they may have been given in too small dosage.

  Side effects are numerous with antibiotics, but usually not severe. That doesn't mean they should be given so indiscriminately as they are today. Antibiotics are commonly prescribed prophylactically (preventively) in all sorts of situations as well as for supposed viral conditions where even the "experts" say they do no good.

  From the get-go, steroids (cortisones by many names) are particularly destructive to important body cells which are necessary for body defense and immune function. This is well known. Still, they are usually prescribed to counteract the body's "inflammatory response," which after almost two centuries of scientific study is still not well understood. Since we don't really understand inflammation after all these years, it seems strange that physicians are so ready and eager to use steroids which essentially interfere with quite normal and common body reaction.

  Second, "If some is good, more is better." Not only are these medications prescribed freely, their dosages are often excessive and time of use can be extended sometimes indefinitely. Clearly with steroids, the longer they are taken the more serious the potential side effects such as depression of immune response, disturbance of bone metabolism, and interference with glandular function. In many situations, "The cure becomes worse than the illness."

  Third, "If all else fails, don't forget the antibiotics and steroids." It is common medical thought that no one should die without the benefits of these two magic bullets. Cortisone and antibiotics are often given in this "shotgun" manner. In fact, much of medicine is played out like target practice with a shotgun. Shotgun medicine is just another name for guesswork.

Is there real magic in these medications? Many will claim that to be the case, and say such has been proven. A Frugal Physician knows that the real magic lies within the patient. "Our remedies oft in ourselves do lie." (William Shakespeare)

The future will see thoughtful medics and Frugal Physicians rethinking the extravagant use of drugs in medical practice and life. Such thoughts will not be new, but resurrected from thinkers like Oliver Wendell Holmes, Sr. (1809-1894).

If this great American physician were to sit in a modern clinic, he would be pleased by many improvements in medical practice. But, I doubt very much that he would take back these famous words: "Throw out opium, which the Creator himself seems to prescribe, for we often see the scarlet poppy growing in the cornfields, as if it were foreseen that wherever there is hunger to be fed there must also be a pain to be soothed; throw out a few specifics which our art did not discover, and it is hardly needed to apply; throw out wine, which is a food, and the vapors which produce the miracle of anesthesia, and I firmly believe that if the whole materia medica [medical drugs], as now used, could be sunk to the bottom of the sea, it would be all the better for mankind, — and all the worse for the fishes." (*Medical Essays*)

Surely, Dr. Holmes would make exceptions for a few more recently developed medications. But on the whole, he would likely consider that modern pharmaceuticals continue to be ineffective, to have frequent side effects, and to often be more detrimental than the problems for which they are prescribed.

Cut to Cure

If drugs form the right arm of modern medicine, surgery makes up the left. The left is surely not as busy as the right arm or half as muscular, but not for the lack of trying. Modern surgeons evolved from the barber-dentist-bonesetters of the past and thus have taken second place to their drug-dealing brother medics. But, they stand proud of their abilities. Surgeons often come to the rescue to bail out their "pill-pushing" fellows in many emergencies.

Surgeons have an aura about them, generally macho and aggressive, in a hurry, no nonsense. Even they have changed with the litigious bent of modern society. Overall, surgeons have had to slow their pace, follow more protocols and bow to more paperwork to be sure that all tests are ordered and Is dotted and Ts crossed.

Early on in medical training, students become aware of the differences between medical specialists: Family physicians are the frontline medics who deal with routine aches and pains. Internists (internal medicine) are the thinkers in medicine who thrive on testing and detective work on difficult problems. Pediatricians are internists in miniature. Obstetrics (and gynecology) is a branch of surgery (more or less), but its practitioners who work constantly with women seem generally more mellow and compassionate. Pathologists and radiologists stand on the fringe of medicine and, it seems, at an even greater distance from people. Most of them rarely get close to patients. Radiologists study Xrays and scans while pathologists read tissue slides and examine corpses. Both are generally aloof from real patient involvement. Psychiatrists study behaviors, often from behind a desk and substantially removed from their patients. They commonly relegate counseling to psychologists and rely on medications to deal with the patients' mind-brains from the physical-chemical angle.

The long white medical frock, which is almost synonymous with medicine and physician-hood has come to symbolize separation: separate knowledge and power as well the separation between physician and patient. These days, physicians are clean and sterile (interesting word - sterile), as if patients are unclean and infectious and dangerous.

Within medicine as a whole, an aphorism circulates which may put some perspective on the various disciplines. It has a number of variations. The following one is typical: "Family physicians know nothing and do nothing. Internists know everything and do nothing. Surgeons know nothing and do everything."

The adage does justice to none of the specialties, yet it gives valuable hints about how they are perceived. It also tends to empower surgeons. Not that they need more.

During the surgical rotation of my internship, I spent much of my time following, assisting, and listening to Dr. Elwood Owens. Owens was a large man and looked bigger when he briskly toured the wards in his white, flowing coat. He had dark hair, a round face, and wore spectacles.

The glasses weren't Army issue. Owens had no intention of looking or acting military any more than required. Elwood was a blunt, talkative, proud Southerner. He really was a "good ol' boy," an enthusiastic operator with eyes on advanced training in cardio-thoracic surgery at Emory University in Atlanta.

He couldn't tell me often enough in his Georgian accent about his plans: "I'm gettin' outa here as soon as I can. I'm gonna do hots (meaning hearts)." Arrogant and obnoxious though he could be, it was hard not to like Owens and get a chuckle from his stories - or at least his telling of them.

One of his favorite ditties went like this: "When the Army drafted me, they made me a Major doing General Surgery. I tried to tell them, 'I would much rather you make me a General doing Major Surgery.'"

Although Dr. Owens tried to maintain an aura of superiority, his impression of himself was not universally shared. Prior to my arrival at Martin Army Hospital, the staff had included another surgeon named Haywood Owens, Elwood's brother. I gathered that Haywood was more productive and less verbal than his younger brother. Tall, red-haired, and good-looking, Haywood favorably impressed many hospital workers. From time to time, the two surgeon-brothers would be seen walking the hospital hallways. A common refrain heard at the time was,

"There they go: Redwood and Deadwood."

Elwood was convinced that surgeons were not only the real elite of the medical profession but also God's greatest gifts to humanity. To become a cardiac surgeon would place him in the highest exalted state. Elwood didn't think much of internists or most other non-surgeons. Speaking with his round, pompous drawl he used to say, "They just play with their tests and pills. Especially those neurologists. Tests and pills. When they get stuck, they have to call on us. We can do anything an internist can do and cut besides. You know that surgery is the only permanent way to cure. We surgeons cut to cure. Yes, we do. Cut to cure."

Surgery is warranted in many situations, especially in the event of trauma. But like the prescription of medication, surgical procedures are much overdone. "My feeling is that somewhere around ninety percent of surgery is a waste of time, energy, money and life." (Robert Mendelsohn)

And, it doesn't take long for a keen observer to discover that cutting does not make for a sure cure even when indications seem clear. In fact, surgery can do more harm than good, especially when entered into precipitately.

"CUT TO CURE," Owens believed.

There are a number of ways to address that idea:

• First, we might want to consider the difference between curing and healing. There is a difference, you know.

Curing is about fixing and repairing. Curing is more superficial, to my way of thinking, than healing. Some ailments can be cured, yet a healing does not take place.

In recent years, different US government administrations have been working to "fix" the medical system. Something like a cure. But, it will take more than "fixes" to put Humpty Dumpty back together again. People are the same. The superficial patching up of patients never guarantees that the effort will be a whole success.

- There may be something to the idea a friend once told me, "You can cure hams, but can't cure people."

The sentiment points to the requirement for the patient - at some level - to be actively involved in the process. Just cutting - even technically perfect, may only take care of one layer of a problem. Human problems almost always are several layers deep. The physical body alone certainly has many layers, but how many others are there yet for scientists and physicians to uncover?

- Another friend, Benjamin Franklin is noted for saying, "God cures and the doctor takes the fee." This idea draws in those layers. It also clearly suggests that the physician's role often may be secondary or even merely window dressing to the healing power of nature.

- Have you ever noticed that "curing" one problem brings another to the surface. That seems to be a common event in home repair. Before you get the original job done, you have created more to deal with than you started. The same thing happens in writing and "curing" a book. It seems next to impossible to edit a book or even an essay to be errorless. Only God is perfect, and I wonder about that some times.

Just think how much more complicated a human being is compared to a book or a home improvement project.

- A Simple incision into the human body is more involved than Regular Surgeons know or will lead their patients to believe. It is not like cutting a cooked ham or turkey which may be a chore in itself.

Cutting into living tissue is like entering a temple. Full preparations and obeisance to holy rites should be followed. (See Holy Presence.) That would go far beyond surgical scrubs and draping. Playing rock and roll in the operating theater is probably not compatible with treating the body as the holy temple which it is. The surgeon's work is most certainly a highly technical skill. Yet, humans are not just biological machines and surgeons obviously need many skills which go far beyond cutting and debriding, excising and sewing.

My mind now carries me back to the Surgery Service at the Hermann Hospital, Houston, Texas. The first surgical patient I met was an elderly black man named Abraham Johnson. He had been in the Surgical Intensive Care Unit for some days and was being readied for skin grafting. Abraham had suffered severe burns to large areas of both legs as the result of a freak accident.

One evening, Abraham had been sitting peacefully in his easy chair watching a favorite television program when his TV exploded before his eyes. Unfortunately, Mr. Johnson had some neurological deficit which prevented him from responding rapidly to this emergency. What should have been a minor mishap became a major physical trauma.

On that same day, we newbies were introduced to the real oddity of the whole surgical wing, Jeremy Jones. Jeremy was a twenty-five year old man who had been injured in a motor vehicle accident several years previously which left him with all of his extremities paralyzed (quadriplegic). Jeremy reacted to his grievous injury by acting out his anger against everyone who came into his aura. He eventually landed in a nursing home. His condition and care deteriorated over time as the aides and nurses "burnt out" trying to deal with both his devastated body and his hostile attitude.

Jeremy had been admitted to the University Hospital because of huge gaping, oozing, stinking bed sores over both hips. He had been treated with the gamut of surgical debridement, continuous dressing changes, and a host of antibiotics with no lasting benefit. The surgical staff was at that time making the decision to do a radical operative procedure to "fix" his problem.

Radical surgical repairs or even routine operations were never (at least in this lifetime) high on my list of favorite medical interests. Oh, there is a genuine mystique about the Operating Room, but not one powerful enough to hold my attention long.

I tried watching surgeries from the operating theater gallery, looking over the shoulders of physicians, nurses, and students in the OR suite, and even peering into the operative field while holding retractors. But, I never obtained much of a view through the surgical incisions or became truly curious regarding the surgeon's prowess.

I was occasionally called upon to hold retractors and considered that task engrossingly boring (another oxymoron). It could be exhausting to stand utterly immobile for what seemed like hours on end doing the job of a very dumb machine - holding a hooked metal bar or two ever so steadily and with the right amount of tension. All too often the surgeon decided that, "You're not holding the retractor firmly enough" or "Damn it, loosen up. You'll tear the guy's flesh." It didn't take long for my feet, back, and eyes to begin to ache. I would selfishly, but unashamedly, pray that the surgeon would work rapidly and efficiently. Fortunately, I was never delegated the job of retracting for one of their marathon procedures. In fact, my retracting days were relatively few as a student as well as an intern. Thank God for small favors. As far as I was concerned, they could take those darn retractors and . . .

Some days along the way, Mr. Johnson was taken to the OR. His legs were grafted with split thicknesses of pig skin in hopes of stimulating recovery from his burns. He was then returned to the SICU for observation. At about the same time, Jeremy's festering wounds had received maximum medical management and his op day also arrived. When the procedure began, there were more techs, students, nurses, and interns in the OR than I could count.

Jeremy was wheeled into the suite on a stretcher and moved to the operating table. The crew not so dexterously propped him on his left side, anesthetized, surgically scrubbed, and draped him. His wounds were still so ugly and wet and pussy that the antiseptic scrub didn't seem likely to have much effect. The surgeons and helpers proceeded to flay his right leg, disarticulate the femur at the hip joint, and create a large pad over the hip with a generous portion of thigh tissue. Bluntly put, they cut his damn leg off!

I managed to watch the spectacle for a half hour or so, but could take only so much. The operation was so revolting to me and my sensibilities. I was equally disturbed by the surgeons simplistic assumption that cutting his leg off would be a quick and effective way to get rid of his "infected" bed sore. Even before he went into surgery, they were making plans to later amputate the other limb.

Despite his terrible physical disability, his emaciated frame, and depressed mental state, Jeremy must have had some powerful will to live. For, he was soon out of intensive care and on a surgical floor. We made regular rounds to dress his surgical wound and the bed sore on his other hip. I always joined rounds. But from that surgery on, I made myself as scarce as possible in the OR.

Mr. Johnson didn't fare as well as Jeremy. Actually, his life was soon in danger for the second time. Mere hours after his grafting, he was spiking a fever, his blood pressure was drifting south, and he was in deep trouble. Johnson was in a state of shock, source undetermined. The surgeons started doing blood cultures, pumping shotgun antibiotics, and pouring in IV meds to prop up his low blood pressure.

Yet, they scratched their heads in wonderment about the cause of the episode. It took several hours of fighting a battle with septic shock before the chief resident had the sense to take a look at the obvious source of the problem -- the recent porcine skin grafts. A grisly, oozing mess appeared when Abraham's dressings were removed. The combination of tissues had become a culture medium and the graft was rejected - or was it the other way around?

With the removal of the dressings and grafts, the cleansing of the slimy debris, and the administration of lots of IV fluids, Abraham came around rapidly. But, the dangers to his recovery were not yet dismissed.

A few days further along, Jeremy was making an amazing recovery. His surgical wound was closing and drainage decreasing. He still had the gaping sore on the opposite hip, but improvement on the surgical side was easily recognizable. He perked up psychologically as well, communicated and cooperated. I remember last seeing him in a wheelchair in the hospital hallway in the center of a conversation. Positive, hopeful attention had effect.

The surgeons seemed to take the results of Jeremy's surgery as some sort of universal sign. One morning, we rounded the SICU and passed beyond Mr. Johnson's bed. The staff talked about their success with Jones and lack thereof with Mr. Johnson. The chief resident was so thrilled with Jeremy's speedy recovery that he couldn't resist, "Maybe we could do Johnson a favor and cure him too by cutting his legs off."

Admittedly, that comment may have "just come out" and was never seriously considered. Still, I just couldn't help but wonder... I soon passed on to another rotation and have no knowledge of eventual outcomes for Misters Jones and Johnson.

Regardless, some surgeons have this simplistic "cut-to-cure" perspective. They sincerely believe they are specially trained and ordained to do "miracles." And, the public clearly buys into their beliefs, spiel, and implied promises. Even though, they never make guarantees.

Wise Physicians and Prudent Patients realize that there is much more to life than the bodies in which we navigate the planet. That even in the 21st century, much is left to be learned about even the material form, which is just the tip of the iceberg of our being. That life and death, coming into and departing the body is always more involved than a medical operation or decision. That real cures - healings - cannot be done to a patient. Such events arise from the inside out. If a physician or surgeon is involved, s/he is just one part of the picture.

Fighting Disease, Saving Lives

A dozen years ago while living in a tiny town (pop. 175) in Montana, I organized a monthly get-together as a way for some people to share their ideas and interests and others to network. The Friday Forum drew 10 to 20 into the parlor of my house at 123 Main Street for presentations on a variety of topics.

I invited one outspoken cowboy, who came back home most summers from Arizona, to "tell us what you think." It took a little persuading to convince him to lead a forum, but just a little. Lester led a provocative meeting based on his question: "Is all of life a play for power?"

You might be able to guess what Lester thought. Most of his audience was agin' his obvious stance. Lester spent much of the program defending his ideas. He did inevitably mention the word "love" once or twice by the time his talk was up.

Lester was a short, moustachioed, hardtack wrangler who hoofed around under a big cowboy hat which made him look that much shorter. Some folks thought he had the Little Man Syndrome (not a medical diagnosis) and spent much of his life trying to stand taller in the saddle. He reminded me a bit of the cartoon character, Yosemite Sam.

He had been married three times, played around more than a bit, but was finally settled with a bright, gentle, accepting school teacher for the previous decade. In a couple revealing moments, he declared to me, "You only have to tell a woman you love her once. That should be more than enough."

Lester was from North Dakota where love can be an unspoken but powerful force in a man's life. His ideas on love reminded me of another North Dakotan and a favorite little story that he told. The funny little man was a Norwegian dairy farmer who smiled and snickered between each sentence of the retelling. He said, "There was this old Norske who loved his wife so much. He practically worshiped the dirt that she walked on. She made the sun rise and set for him. Oh, he just adored her. He loved her so much, he ALMOST told her."

Well, Lester told his lady friend once, or so he said. Maybe he just imagined he had. Love was obviously not a big part of his vocabulary or his way of doing business. Power was the key for him. And, that was not likely to change. We know it is hard for the leopard to change its spots and equally so for an old Scorpionic, Germanic North Dakotan, dusty cowpoke.

It is hard for any of us to change even when we want to - or think we want to. Patterns are tough to bend within people, in systems, in countries and in the whole world. The ways of medicine, being part of systems and the rest of the world, are no different.

Much of medical practice is predicated on control, which is just another name for power. The patient hands over his/her power to a physician; patients and physicians empower drugs and surgery as their front line and rearguard forces in cases of illness and injury; the medical establishment monopolizes control of health and disease concerns in the western world; a hierarchy rules within all medical facilities; etc..

The importance of power is seen quite obviously in the medical system in the never-ending need to -

Combat disease.	Turn the tide of battle.
Fight the good fight.	Beat it.
Cut it out.	Kill those germs.
Destroy the invaders.	Ward off attack.
Reinforce with more antibiotics.	Boost the armamentarium.

We do indeed FIGHT disease, because we make it out to be the enemy. This is the prevailing model and has been so practically forever. The medical model, which sets the bar for many of the other limited options in the modern world, tends to see most any human discomfort, pain, aberration as disease which must be expunged, dissipated or conquered at all costs.

This is unwritten law and Regular Physicians rarely stop to think that there may be more than a few holes in such wide-ranging and potent belief. Though change comes hard, this simplistic approach must be transformed as more enlightened perspectives come to the fore in medicine and modern thinking in general.

Actually, "new" thinking is often just a reappearance of ancient wisdom. For, "there is nothing new under the sun." (Ecclesiastes) Alternative views, albeit sometimes esoteric, have been and continue to be held the world around. The greatest of hoary teachings have not made their way into the common curricula or standard practice. In part because such a step will require more than concrete ability and mechanical thinking.

The following story comes out of ancient Korean Zen tradition. The teaching behind the story can and will have widespread application in medical circles when the focus of medicine shifts from its current bases of body, disease and fighting to higher levels.

"One morning as he is getting dressed, the hard-working prince of a powerful kingdom notices two red, painful spots on his thigh. Assuming them to be the bites of a poisonous insect that had burrowed into the royal bedclothes, he scolds his chamberlain, orders the silk sheets burned, and without a second thought begins his routine of palace duties.

"But later that night, readying himself for bed, the prince beholds a chilling sight: The two bumps on his leg have turned into a pair of curiously darting eyes! Only with great difficulty he goes into a fitful sleep. The minute dawn breaks, he flings aside his coverlets to inspect his leg. To his horror, not only are the eyes still there, but now, beneath them, a pair of rhythmically flaring nostrils! Terrified lest anyone discover his affliction, he binds his leg with a silken bandage; ignoring the faint sound of labored breathing (the nose seems to inhale each time he does), he attends to the affairs of state.

"That evening, at a ceremonial banquet for his vassal-warlords from the outlying districts, he makes a pretense of merriment. But the assembled guests are startled by a muffled shout from beneath the table. The prince clamps his hand over his leg, nearly losing two of his fingers in the process: His symptom has grown a mouth!

"Hastily excusing himself in the ensuing hubbub, he runs at full tilt to his private quarters, summons the court surgeon and, swearing him to silence, forces him to operate and cut away the face. A miracle cure!

"For several months, life returns to normal. But one day, as the prince leads his elite horse cavalry in a wheeling close-order drill, a furious scream erupts from nowhere: His symptom has returned with a vengeance. The prince's mount shies and rears, landing him in the mud. His men, hearing the secret face's strange cries, break ranks. Rumors begin to fly through the capital that the ruler is possessed by demons.

"A second clandestine operation is performed, and a third, but to no avail. The face relentlessly reappears. Now unable to leave his room, the prince spends his days receiving magi and astrologers, muttering old frauds all, while the kingdom falls into disarray. Finally a grizzled monk in frayed saffron robes barges unannounced into the prince's chambers. Brushing aside the hand-wringing courtiers, he informs the prince of a stream that lies off in a corner of a distant province, protected by Kwan Yin, the goddess of compassion. Its miraculous waters heal all wounds.

Equipped with the monk's scrawled map, the prince sets out with a small company of imperial horsemen. After an arduous journey -- during which the face, despite being swaddled in layers of muslin, continues its loud, inarticulate bawling -- the party arrives at the sacred stream. Eagerly the prince leaps from his horse and removes a silver chalice from his gold-embroidered saddlebag.

"He unwraps his leg and is about to pour the holy water on the hated face to silence it forever, when its mouth stops shouting. 'Wait!' it cries out. 'All this time, you have never even looked closely at me nor tried to understand a single word I have said. Do you not recognize me?'

"The prince, gazing closely, suddenly recognizes a distorted likeness of his own face, its eyes filled with a pain long unacknowledged. At the sight of it, the prince begins to weep, and as he does so the face begins to soften, the eyes growing limpid, melting into those of Kwan Yin herself. 'You had no heart of compassion,' she says. 'No sword of self-insight. How else could I summon you to your true nature?' Now the courtiers, decamped at a curious distance, heard the sound of two voices talking, long into the night, about the secret suffering that had been disturbing the prince's sleep long before the face had appeared. When the sun came up, the prince had been healed – though a single eye would occasionally reappear and look around, just as a reminder."

(This story is retold by Marc Ian Barasch in *The Healing Path*. Barasch's book is one of the best available on the subject of healing whether written by layperson or physician.)

This story and the common pattern of Fighting Disease should give us pause to reflect on some simple, straightforward questions. Ones that Frugal Physicians naturally ponder. These queries help him/her put illness and injury into the framework of the rest of life.

• Are symptoms, illnesses, disease foreign to nature? Are they mistakes? Or, part of the course of life?
• Are humans part of nature? Is nature prone to error?
• How can fighting diseases of which we REALLY DON'T KNOW

the causes ever be truly successful?
- What are the REAL effects of fighting battles inside the human body? When we are only guessing?
- Are there better ways?

Way back when I met Dr. Smythe and heard him talk about the importance of a physician's history and examination over testing, another keen point of interest arose during those medical rounds.

Like all stories, there are two sides to this one. Both need to be heard. You generally get Dr. Booth's side. Today, you get my side. The word had spread about the hospital halls that Dr. David Booth, the other resident on St. Joseph's Internal Medicine Service, had recently resuscitated a patient. Code Blue had been called.

Booth came to the rescue and brought the patient back to life.

The incident came up on rounds and Booth got his just due. While he gloated a bit, Dr. Smythe moved on to discuss the importance of technical skill versus sympathetic care.

While I had never run a code or "retrieved" a life until that time, I had to speak up for being human and compassionate with our patients and not just technicians. "Medical skills only go so far. Quality of life is important to every one."

Booth and others trumped what little I dared to say with, "You gotta keep 'em alive. You can give them all the sympathy you want. But, if your patient dies, what good have you done?"

My experience was limited then and would never be as great in that area of medicine. So, I have to grant Dr. Booth his point or, at least, some of it.

Here are other angles from which to view the issue:

- I think it bears saying again and again, "Death is inevitable and unavoidable, even for physicians." Medics believe their calling is to relieve suffering and keep disease and death at bay. But, one skill a Frugal Physician develops while getting to really know his/her patients is to get a sense of their time-line - one that can add quality to breath and heartbeat.

This has surely gotten harder to determine in a natural sort of way as people move more frequently, change doctors, go to specialists and subspecialists. One of the values of having a family or general practitioner is the potential of seeing the same health care provider for decades, if not generations.

A Wise Physician accepts death as a part of the cycles of life. S/he uses life-saving measures selectively and understands that death is ultimately part of everyone's healing process.

- During my internship days, I remember one day when Dr. Ed and I were acting as MODs (Medical Officers of the Day). We had heard that a seriously ill patient was being transported to the hospital, but that was it. No details. No diagnosis. No word as to who his regular physician may have been.

All of a sudden, we got paged to the Intensive Care Unit, "MOD Stat." In flowing white coats we appeared and found a sad situation. A dying or dead man lying on a litter with tubes and equipment and people all around waiting to be put into action to "save his life."

His heart had stopped beating, but that wasn't all. His face was bloated, belly hugely distended. His whole body was yellow. And, he had bloody vomitus smeared around his mouth and chest.

Dr. Ed and I stared at each other, "What have we walked into?" To resuscitate or not to resuscitate was the question.

But, we just couldn't jump in. As far as we were concerned, "Even if we can resuscitate him, his body appears to be shot."

To the eventual consternation of a few, we decided to call our patient, "Dead on Arrival." There was some fallout, at least gossip about it. But, no one could really fault us much because, "They weren't there in our shoes with a Dead Man and no information suggesting he had any potential to return to life with an adequate body." Raising the dead can and has been done, but surely is not always warranted.

- Since leaving medicine, I have encountered a small number of people who have been resuscitated. The only ones who have spoken about their experience, said, "It was the worst thing that ever happened to me. I would rather have died. I swear, they will never do that to me again."

Those recountings chimed in with some, but not all the people I encountered who went through similar moments in my medical days. In both time periods, they were older people with major medical problems. Context is clearly important. But certainly, not everyone whose heart stops with medical professionals around should be put through the resuscitation ordeal.

- The coming of the age of electrical defibrillators brings forth the programmed command to some people, "We won't let you die without the benefit of a few whopping jolts of electricity. Here comes!" There are many cases when efforts at resuscitation are warranted. But, probably many more incidents occur in which CPR (Cardio-Pulmonary Resuscitation) is questionable.

Medical studies clearly suggest that when someone's heart stops beating, professionals only have a few minutes (5 to 10) to get an effort going to even have a chance at successful resuscitation.

- Even in the best of situations with all the equipment around and trained personnel ready, the odds of CPR being successful are very low. Yet, crash carts and defibrillators are becoming more and more visible beyond the hospital and clinic settings.

There has been a push in recent years to install electrical defibrillators in malls and ballparks, etc. So if someone tries to die, s/he can be shocked back to life by anyone who comes along and can read directions.

Although the makers of these machines may be well intentioned, one can't help but question the validity of this practice. And wonder about the financial factor. All those defibrillators spreading around the western world add up to lots of income for some.

Even then, the premise to "save lives" may be simple. But, there is a rub, or two, in the equation. The element of time, the need to read directions, the "stage" for the event, etc.

It is hard enough to get someone to work a fire extinguisher properly the first time. A scary situation. But, nothing like trying to bring a dead person back to life using an alien device in a strange place at the spur of the moment. Undoubtedly, some people are getting shocked in malls whose hearts are just fine. At least before they get zapped.

In the present era, physicians are convincing patients that the inevitable can be forestalled. Many patients are walking around with Implantable Cardioverter-Defibrillators (ICDs). If their heart starts to fibrillate, the device automatically gives them a "healthy" dose of electricity. The device says, "I won't let you die."

- My singular "life-saving" effort occurred in the obstetrical unit of Martin Army Hospital. I had just delivered the infant son of an unmarried woman. There had been no particular problems during her pregnancy nor during the course of her labor. (If there had, the staff obstetrician would have likely done the honors or been standing over the shoulder of his intern.)

The child arrived and gave a brief, but forceful cry. His color was good and everything fine. But, within seconds the infant stopped breathing. A potential catastrophe was on my hands. However, from that moment everything moved as if planned and choreographed.

One nurse attended the mother and another carried the infant to the lighted warming table in the corner of the delivery suite. A third nurse prepared a laryngoscope and an endotracheal tube. In a trice, I positioned the child's head, inserted the laryngoscope blade through his vocal cords, and placed the tube into his trachea. A nurse connected an airbag to the tube and gave the baby a few puffs of air. By the time the staff man arrived, the infant was breathing and bellering normally on his own.

That instant reinforced an element of my growing medical philosophy. It seemed to me that despite the scare, that child was meant to live. I remember running through the motions of intubating the newborn as if someone or something was working through me. I seemed to perform the procedure as an accomplished technician, but I had had only two previous experiences of intubation under my belt. Both of them were under controlled circumstances in the operating room. I had been guided through the process ahead of two adult surgical cases during medical school. An anesthesiologist had directed my eyes and hands in both instances. In the real life emergency, I also felt myself guided, almost pushed through the procedure, by a quite invisible mentor.

I feel comfortable with my conclusion, based on that and other medical moments, that physicians don't really save or heal anyone. We are not doing the REAL work.

Physicians are at best channels - important and necessary though they can be - for the true healing forces which are not apparent to our usual senses. It is my distinct sense that physicians and nurses can't cause the shortening of a person's life by simple error - the patient's time must have arrived.

I firmly believe that we are protected from pain, injury and death which does not rightfully belong to us. Furthermore, health and welfare are also determined by forces much, much greater than those ordained at graduation from medical school.

PART II: ENTHUSIASM

Medical Heresy

Dr. Robert Mendelsohn was an unorthodox thinker and writer. Highly credentialed, but little heeded, Mendelsohn was The Frugal Physician of the 70s and 80s. He was very critical of the medical system in general and of pediatric practice, obstetrics with its predominance of male obstetricians, and vaccination in particular. He featured himself to be a "medical heretic" and wrote *Confessions of a Medical Heretic* as well as *Male Practice: How Doctors Manipulate Women and How To Raise a Healthy Child In Spite of Your Doctor*. Mendelsohn was a pediatrician like Dr. Benjamin Spock, but of the renegade, iconoclastic type.

Drawing on his twenty-five years in active medical practice, Mendelsohn became convinced that -

- Annual physical examinations are a health risk.
- Hospitals are a dangerous place for the sick.
- Most operations do little good and many do harm.
- Medical testing laboratories are scandalously inaccurate.
- Many drugs cause more problems than they cure.
- The Xray machine is the most pervasive and most dangerous tool in the doctor's office.

Major inaccuracies of laboratory testing have not been this writer's experience. But, most of Mendelsohn's other assertions seem correct. Thirty years haven't changed many medical practices for the better.

Maybe, it is time for more heretics to simply state that there are better ways to deal with medical ills in America and the world. Change and improvements are possible and clearly needed.

- We can reduce medical care costs.
- We can expand options for care beyond the usual monopoly.
- We can take a breather from technological adventures.

- We can look more at individuals than protocols and statistics.
- We can put more compassion into care.
- We can work more at understanding problems than fixing them.
- We can look at health and disease, living and dying holistically.
- We can make room in our lives for disease and healing.
- We can consider that humans are more than flesh, bone and blood.

The Medical Heretic would most assuredly support such thinking if he were still around in the 21st century. He would surely note the growing effects of the Medical Industrial Complex, pharmaceutical propaganda, surgical implants and chronic drug use, astronomical costs, assembly line care, etc.

There is one heresy which Dr. Mendelsohn did not broach and likely would leave unspoken even in the present medical climate: Most of the touted advances and benefits of modern medicine are simply illusions. I repeat, "The supposed benefits of medicine are largely illusions."

Put simply, "The sick and injured generally recover or not in similar time frames with or without intervention." It's just a broader version of getting over the flu in a week (7 days) with or without medicine. The major difference arises in the costs - financial and otherwise - to you, the patient.

The reader won't want to even consider the possibility that this large generalization could be true unless I add: There are exceptions to every rule, a small percentage. You undoubtedly know of some. "Nothing is totally true and even that is not totally true." (Multatuli)

A story seems to fit here. Dr. Dan (see Purple Pills) took me to a meeting of one of the study groups that he frequented. I was not keen on going, but the session turned out to be congenial. It was a smiley gaggle of middle-agers, almost all females, led by a respected business man in his 50s and held at his home. John, the host, garnered extra attention leading a group of older folks and being practically the only man at most sessions.

The topic was *A Course in Miracles*. I had studied the Course several years previously, attended other groups, and even led one on my own. That put me at an advantage - I knew the material. And a disadvantage

- I probably knew too much. Or, thought I did.

I also was aware through Dan that John had been having health problems and attending medical providers. He was diagnosed with leukemia and was in the process of "taking the cure."

Illusion is one of the recurring themes in *A Course in Miracles*. Our attachments and beliefs being major illusions which prevent us from living more fully, changing our perceptions of the world, and experiencing the "miracles" of life. Things just aren't really as they appear and as we wish them to be. And, that's much of what brings us pain, anger, fear and loss.

Recurring and repeated comments were made that evening on "This is an illusion," and, "Oh, that belief is an illusion." Just before a break, medicine came up in the conversations a number of times. Medicine being sacrosanct, no one dared say or imagine the obvious about it. No one but I.

I couldn't help myself, raised my hand, and suggested something like, "I know this may be hard for some people to hear. But, medicine and our belief in it is as much an illusion as many other parts of life that we hold onto so tightly."

That turned out to be a good time for the break. Nothing more was said of medicine as an illusion. Nor did I return to the group meeting to bring the idea up again.

The first part of this book pointed out medicine's problems many of which can be dealt with through simple common sense. But, there are layers and layers. This second section will attempt to peel back a few deeper layers so that we can peek beyond the bodily illusion. This should provide hints about our real natures and potentials for healing.

Hopefully, this approach will give Frugal Physicians, patients and the reader things to get enthusiastic about. It has done that for the writer.

Good Medicine, Bad Medicine

Despite obvious and common shortcomings, modern medicine has indeed done some amazing things during its development over the last several generations. Those advances are just a beginning. It is hard to imagine what the state of medicine will be hundreds of years from now. But, it will be built on some of the accomplishments of recent history.

Even now, medical care excels in some areas while others lag far behind those in which technology and common sense come to the rescue. We don't want to "throw out the baby with the bath water." Let's first look at positive points in medicine - where medicine excels and where consumers can expect real benefits.

- First Aid. This tops them all. In case of true emergency, access to a Trauma Center puts patients in the best possible position for immediate, skilled and effective treatment. "If doctors reduced their involvement with people by ninety percent and attended only emergencies, there's no doubt in my mind that we'd be better off." (Robert Mendelsohn)

Medicine, like most disciplines, does its best work in situations where problems are clear and well-defined. That is usually the case in true emergencies. If you have one, you want to be near a tried and trusty big city ER.

In motor vehicle injuries, construction mishaps, explosions, gun shot wounds and the like, life threatening problems can be quickly assessed and substantive care provided. Operating theaters and intensive care units can be mobilized to support body functions for extended periods. This is television *ER* at work doing its finest. If medicine ever "saves lives," it is in such settings.

- Man-made injuries. From another angle, medicine is best in dealing with problems which human advancement and technology have helped to create. Like wounds from bullets, moving vehicles, and falling objects. If human beings created the implement of injury, they have likely prepared - to some degree - for the sinister effects of such products and structures.

Many, many modern medical innovations have come out of the effects of warfare. Every new weapon has spawned new medical advances to deal with man's aggression. Military medics and surgeons have literally been at the front lines to deal with new kinds of injuries as well as their long term effects. Warfare has obviously damaging effects. It also has the effect of creating products and procedures which help civilians in peace time. Prosthetic limbs, skin grafting, cosmetic repair, joint replacement, etc. have evolved out of War Medicine.

There are numerous drawbacks to such advances: The tools and weapons of war have rolled over into civilian life. Wounds from AK47s don't just occur on battlefields. Cosmetic surgery becomes a fetish with some. Joint replacement has become commonplace, routine and excessive.

- Prosthesis. Centuries removed from barbaric amputations and equally crude prostheses (wooden legs), surgeons have become proficient at removing and replacing limbs. The former aided by anesthesia and the latter with computers. Those two aspects, however, are only half the battle, so to speak. The body must adapt and adapt. Healing from such major trauma is generally a very long process.

From prosthetic advances have come joint replacements which are more and more common. Orthopedic surgery is a booming business. Surgeons have the aura and patients have the belief that joints are as replaceable as teeth. (Teeth are not all that replaceable.) They forget that even if joint replacement is a "success," they are trading one problem for another. Maybe one problem for several.

Every bodily intervention has wide ranging effects. Some take months or years to show, as in the taking of medication. Some of the effects are undoubtedly in other body systems. Despite what physicians and scientists suggest, there is no metal or substance which can be implanted in the body which is totally innocuous.

"Bone on bone" (pretty simplistic) is the common refrain - along with patient complaints - which gets people into the operating theater to have their living joints sawn out and titanium ones hammered in. Watching such surgery is like viewing a carpenter in action. But, the bone carpenter is in a hurry, makes a bloody mess, and expects miracles out of his quick work. S/he has only one attempt and fitting opportunities are hardly optimal.

Physicians and patients forget that people are not machines with interchangeable parts. Every human "part" is invested and connected with numerous layers and lines, tissues and vessels, networks and systems - visible and invisible. All much more complicated than any man-made device ever will be.

Every surgical invasion of the body or chemical intervention (medication) has acute AND long term effects. Nonetheless, medics and cutters persist in spreading their trades thinking that they KNOW. How little do THEY know! How little do WE know!

Robert Mendelsohn retold a thought-provoking story which any potential orthopedic surgery patient might wish to ponder: "My favorite example of how doctors can be less intelligent than the situation calls for is a matter of public record. As part of the hearings before the Senate Health Subcommittee, Senator Edward Kennedy recalled a skiing injury to his shoulder, suffered when he was a young man. His father called in four specialists to examine the boy and recommend treatment. Three recommended surgery. The advice of the fourth doctor, who did not recommend surgery, was followed, however. He had just as many degrees as the others. The injury healed. Senator Kennedy's colleagues then proceeded to question Dr. Lawrence Weed, Professor of Medicine at the University of Vermont and originator of a highly popular patient record system for hospitals. Dr. Weed's reply was the 'senator's shoulder probably would have healed as satisfactorily if the operation had been performed.'"

The reader can make his/her own observations on this story. It was and still is quite a shocker to this writer.

• Poisonings. Humans have probably made more poisons in the last hundred years than nature has in eons. Certainly, infinitely more people go to the hospital for artificial poisoning than ones they consume in nature, like mushrooms. Still, if chemists can make a poison, they can also make antidotes. And usually do. So in case of poisoning, deliberate or incidental, "Hie thee to the hospital."

While considering poisoning, it seems appropriate to point out how downright deliberate poisoning so commonly occurs in the medical setting. Practically all of cancer chemotherapy is medical poisoning. If the disease won't kill you, the chemical "cure" has a good chance.

Chemotherapy is meant to poison and destroy the "bad cells" more quickly than the good cells. A neat trick. It may be no more than a trick. But, it certainly is poison, toxic and traumatic to the human system.

I can't help remembering when my mother used to come home from her chemotherapy infusions for breast cancer. The poison was then coursing through her bloodstream into her whole system. Even at a distance, I felt stirred and scared. I reflected on Mom's state, "She's buzzing."

- Restorative surgery. The author has been impressed by the benefits of some surgeries. The list is not long and most of these have obvious and outward effect. Cataract surgery, in which the defective lens of the eye is removed and replaced, is generally very successful and dramatically improves the quality of a person's life.

Cosmetic repair of face and skin after injuries can have profoundly beneficial effects. Some orthopedic repairs like those for congenital deformities can be impressive.

On the other hand, surgical procedures in general are way out of hand. Caesarean sections are sometimes as frequent as one in four deliveries. Something is not quite kosher there.

Tonsillectomies are not as common as they used to be, but still much overdone. Appendectomies should be passe in this age. Hysterectomies are far too readily recommended and performed. Gall bladders are even being removed from children in the present day. What next?!

Some surgical procedures are downright hokum. Modern versions of snake oil. Tennis elbow surgery for one. The operation severs the tendon to supposedly relieve pain. Scientific rationale behind the procedure is non-existent. "But it works." Eventually. And so does time.

Like the cortisone shots which often precede it, the tenotomy is a very common, wasteful, inane procedure. Many rotator cuff operations fit pretty much in the same ballpark. Cutting into healthy functioning tissue to cure a temporary functional problem often causes more of them in the future. As stated earlier, it is amazing what human bodies and systems can tolerate. We are so fortunate that the human form is so wonderfully constructed.

We have taken a quick look at Good Medicine, with more than a few forays into Bad Medicine. Sadly, there is still much of the latter because of our medical ignorance and continued blind belief in medicine as we know it. We must become willing to explore other aspects, layers and dimensions of human life. When we do, Frugal Physicians will be part of that change and help bring in a new era of real knowledge and true health.

Diagnosis, Disease and Dis-ease

The theory and practice of medicine has been based on the concept of diagnosis for centuries. DIAGNOSIS is huge in medicine. Big as it is, it merely amounts to the labeling of combinations of symptoms and signs. That is, giving a NAME to a patient's medical problem.

Physicians believe that they are thus identifying an illness to the exclusion of others which gives them information on how to intervene for the betterment of the patient. The whole process is fraught with problems and shortcomings, errors and illusions.

• Identification. As in IDing (identifying) a youth or a suspect. John Doe and you and the rest of us are quite unique and "identifiable" using simple criteria.

In the case of disease, methods for identifying even the "usual suspects" are rarely cut and dried, simple and straight-forward. Tests have proliferated to a large degree because hardly any are disease-specific. Likewise, hardly any diseases are specific and static. There is rarely one test or finding which makes a diagnosis. "We got our crook. That test just nailed him for sure."

Not so lucky. Thus, one more test. "Oh, we can start you on some medication. But, the last word isn't in yet. These things are quite variable, you know. We think we have it. But, let's check further. In the meantime, we'll try this regimen."

- Illness. Human beings almost always have illnesses, not diseases. Physicians do much better with diseases. And so do patients. Medics are trained and good at treating diseases not people.

The difference between illness and disease arises because people respond to stresses - external and internal, physical and emotional and financial and mental and social and spiritual - in innumerable ways. "One man's poison is another man's meat." Quite truly so. Some extraordinary persons can swallow Skull and Crossbones poisons with absolutely no effect. Others have adverse, sometimes fatal, responses to a peanut chip or a whiff of perfume.

Why did John Doe have a major reaction to a peanut butter cookie or a piece of shrimp? Regular Physician's answer: "Well, he obviously had an anaphylactic reaction. You know, allergens and histaminic responses and all that stuff." That hardly answers the question, but we too often accept such Regular Medicine talk as scientific and valid. Medical jargon is often merely descriptive, pseudo-scientific, and/or simply deceptive.

The stressor is thus not the main factor in creating illness. Disease-causing agents are all around and within us. But, illness only happens to certain people, at certain times, and under certain conditions. An "allergic reaction" is an illness, not a disease.

- Exclusion. Much of medical practice is spent not just on diagnosis, but on differential diagnosis. This is often where the bills mount up. On the first round, a handful of symptoms, maybe a finding on physical examination, and/or an abnormal test lead a physician to make a list of potential diagnoses. To attempt to "prove" one diagnosis, often a highly intellectual and unnecessary exercise, calls for more testing - and costs.

Rather than really proving, s/he spends time and money trying to Rule Out all but one in the list. Your doctor does not want to treat the wrong disease. Even though s/he may give the same medication and recommendations.

Ruling In and Ruling Out are significant WORDS. They point back to the importance of power and control in the hands of medics. Real or perceived.

- Intervention. We have considered intervention a few times already. The medical protocol leads from identification to intervention (treatment of some kind). Most physician-patient interactions result in some kind of intervention. Easily two thirds lead to prescription medication.

The alternative? How about considering that the symptoms, etc. are part of a natural process. The problem will likely resolve itself as time is a great healer. There may be something worth experiencing which comes with these discomforts. The illness may bring a lesson to be learned. The problem brings its own resolution. The human body is going through a minor internal overhaul. Change is being incubated within. The body is being readied for new function.

These are just a few possible ways in which illness, so-called disease, may be acting in a person's life. Disease may be better left alone. Intervention often adds to the discomfort, turmoil and expense of illness. But, it clearly keeps the patient occupied instead of "just doing nothing and waiting until it's over."

It is well worth noting that medical diagnosis is the sole privilege and responsibility of a licensed physician. Physicians are thus set apart from other providers and the laity. Only they are trained, authorized to make diagnoses, and afforded that power.

While diagnosis sets physicians apart from the crowd, medics use this method to set one disease apart from another. The word diagnosis comes from the Greek. The parts of the word are dia = apart, and gnosis

= knowledge.

Originally, the word meant discerning, discriminating and deciding between two possibilities. In the modern day, diagnosis has taken on a broader meaning which has led to the idea of differential diagnosis as mentioned above.

In fact, the discerning and discriminating abilities of Regular Physicians are themselves rather suspect. The special knowledge (gnosis - the Gnostics were an ancient Christian sect of knowers) which physicians claim has long been guarded, parochial and monopolistic. Regardless of how physicians present and how patients and public perceive their diagnostic abilities, such true knowledge as medics really have is woefully limited.

Nonetheless, diagnosis is fundamental to the concept of disease and the practice of present-day medicine. What would a modern physician do without diagnosis and disease? S/he would be lost at sea, adrift, without oar or paddle.

There are very few Real Diseases. They can be counted on one hand. The rest of human ailments should be looked at from an entirely different angle. Even Real Diseases are not as simple as usually believed.

In all cases of illness and disease, what people really have and take to their physician are complaints and symptoms of which they know little and of which their physician often knows less. Dis-ease is a better term for this state of being.

The idea of dis-ease, which the writer first borrowed from Edgar Cayce, dates back to the days of Hippocrates when physicians were generally more patient oriented. It seems worthy of resurrecting into modern time and practice. If patients and physicians were to consider health concerns first as Dis-ease rather than Disease, a whole new sense of illness might be developed. This would take large bites out of the medical system, laboratory and Xray testing, paperwork and expense. It would also cut away some of the medical mystique, much to the benefit of patient welfare and the detriment of physician authority.

Should doctors think more in terms of dis-ease rather than disease, it would become easier for both to put problems in the larger context of life and experience. Rather than the usual brief history, cursory exam, and review of systems combined with ever expanding test batteries.

Instead of fitting patients into the medical system and diagnostic methods, physicians would really come to know their patients and themselves. They would then also rediscover the teaching of the Father of American Medicine, Sir William Osler: "It is much more important to know what sort of patient has a disease, than what sort of disease a patient has."

Anything Can Cause Anything

However you look at them, so-called diseases are not beings. Physicians and patients turn signs and tests, symptoms and discomfort and dysfunction into creatures which we call disease. When in fact, they are really dealing with dis-ease.

A dis-ease is simply an aberration from our usual way of life. It sure may seem much more than that when we are passing through times of illness and pain. When we get a glimmer of the Bigger Picture, we begin to realize otherwise.

Disease or dis-ease becomes problem and pest, adversary and nemesis, sometimes even our mortal enemy. Often because we as individuals, as physicians, and as the human race lack fundamental understanding of how the human form works and life transpires through it.

Imagine for a moment that you have been experiencing discomfort for days. Maybe headache, nausea, cough, weakness, fatigue. Days become a week; your self treatment, shoddy or otherwise, has been unhelpful. Your symptoms have been getting in the way of doing a good job at work, helping out at home, and being able to enjoy life. You keep pushing until you tell yourself, "Something's wrong with me. I've got some kind of crud. I think I will go to the doctor and find out what's going on."

If your car or home air conditioner were acting up, you would get it checked and repaired or replaced before long. But, they are machines.

All parts are man-made. They were designed by human beings. Chances are quite high that the malfunction could be detected and remedied. A switch, a gizmo, a widget cleaned or repaired and things get back to "normal." Or, as is not uncommon, a few pieces are replaced. "To cover the possibilities. Just in case."

Well, human beings were not designed by humans. New parts are not easy to come by. Actually, there are no new parts. Transplants use old parts which came from a different system. Man-made implants and replacements (like joints) do work, but often not as touted and they do because the human organism is amazingly adaptable. But, those implants wear out and are subject to all sorts of problems which sooner or later become human ones.

If the human being can adapt to an implant, it should be able to adapt to most dis-ease. In fact it does and has for eons. Physicians and medicine have appeared and suggest they have ready answers to whatever ails us. Sorry, that is pretty much a fairy tale.

The situation is especially problematic in the present age. We haven't got the time or understanding to allow the ebb and flow of life to put us down, to throw us in bed, to box our ears. "You're not listening. Time to pay attention. You are getting in your way."

Disease hasn't been manufactured on assembly lines to certain specifications to get our attention. But, life does have ways to make us eventually take notice. C.S. Lewis reminds us that, "God whispers to us in our pleasures, speaks in our conscience, but shouts in our pain."

Unfortunately, our attention is pinpointed on our body or the parts that aren't working up to expectation. If they aren't working like they used to, then there is something wrong and medical intervention is in order. So we believe.

During my first year of medical school, I used to make a weekly (decidedly unofficial) visit to Texas Chiropractic College in nearby Pasadena. My purpose was to broaden my education and learn about the hands-on skills chiropractors were taught. I thought that chiropractors and osteopaths might know some things of which orthodox medicine was ignorant. And they do.

I followed an upper-level chiropractic student in the clinic during my visits, watched him go through the paces, and spend time with his hands on his patients. The chiropractic clinic facility was pretty bare bones, and obviously there wasn't a lot of money flowing into Chiropractic. But, I was impressed that chiropractors have means of access to humans and their bodies that orthodoxy has almost totally overlooked or avoided.

On one trip, I purchased a copy of a book written by Dr. William Harper, the college's president. All I clearly remember today about it is the title: *Anything Can Cause Anything*, one which would attract the attention of hardly any medically trained people, then or now. Dr. Harper wrote his book to reiterate and expand on principles of chiropractic. To restate the "proven" and reenergize the tenets of his profession.

He didn't spend much time on his premise because he was mostly re-proving Chiropractic, which for all its shortcomings, does have an underlying and relatively cohesive philosophy. Regular Medicine doesn't. Chiropractic teaches that a preponderance of illness is caused by subluxation of vertebrae in the spinal column which adversely affect nearby nerves and vessels. Those ill effects spread outward to body parts near and far.

With the book long since read and largely forgotten, I still retain the simple idea stated in its title. Human beings have many similarities, especially in their bodies. But, they have quite singular experiences in health as well as going into dis-ease, moving through it, and coming out the other side.

People develop their dis-ease from a host of different avenues. No two cases of any "disease" are identical. How could they be, even if diseases were fixed? People, including patients, are unique and have unique experiences.

Regular Medicine looks for single specific causes for specific named diseases. It expects that the world, nature, and the body react in set ways to these diseases and respond to treatment as anticipated. Furthermore, Regular Physicians consider their patients more or less one-dimensionally. That dimension is the physical.

Life doesn't play by such simple rules. Human beings are neither simple, nor one-dimensional. Dr. Harper's premise that Anything Can Cause Anything is pretty much true. And, there is the rub for practitioners of any ilk. Even chiros. Anything Can Cause Anything because all things are connected. "All roads lead to Rome," so to speak for ill and good, disease and healing.

Most of medical rules and labels and tabulations and categories fall apart in any single case of any particular dis-ease. However classic that case may be.

Medics use statistics to support their efforts in diagnosis and treatment of all sorts of disease - generally the ones they can pin down with some sort of test. But, most of us know that statistics are limited and subject to manipulation. ("Statistics, damned statistics and lies." Benjamin Disraeli) And in any single case of any disease, statistics are largely meaningless.

Again, we are talking about human beings who have a predisposition to avoiding simple representation in numbers or names. Even the simplest of ailments have so much variation and appear in people's lives for so many reasons. Let's take some examples to give a broad picture of causes of common dis-eases:

• Sore throat - I can give a personal story here, recalling the time I experienced a raging "strep" throat at the end of a long summer trip with a woman friend and her two sons many years ago. The very simple solution - nothing medical was used at all - was a conversation in which we decided to give up plans to consolidate our households and to go our separate ways. My swollen glands, difficulty swallowing, pain and discomfort along with angry red and pustular tonsils disappeared less than 24 hours after we engaged in our "therapeutic" conversation.

Pharyngitis (in medicalese) may appear in people who are talking too much (akin to common thought on laryngitis), patients who can't "swallow" things forced upon them, persons holding back their feelings such that they can't let them out. Sore throat may show in someone who feels like s/he is being strangled or drowned. Or when that part of the anatomy is misused or abused physically or emotionally. In the minds of many Regular Doctors, these may be considered remote influences. Wise Practitioners, searching beyond the surface of things, recognize that they can be much more important that any germ. Even the much maligned *Streptococcus*.

In previous generations, chronic sore throat frequently resulted in a trip to the hospital and a tonsillectomy. That was in the era when children were to be "seen and not heard." The trend has changed decidedly. Let the reader consider the implications of such as we move onto another dis-ease.

In this era, tonsillitis is less common as opposed to otitis media which has become near epidemic. Part of the picture is the change in attitude towards children. Nowadays, youngsters are allowed fuller expression at the same time they "cover their ears and won't listen." To the author, this fits the symptoms which come with otitis media (middle ear infection, so-called).

Earache, like sore throat, is usually treated as a strictly physical problem with decongestants as well as antibiotics. Unless other dimensions are considered, obvious and important causative factors can be easily overlooked.

- Asthma - Volumes are written about asthma which has become an increasingly major problem in modern times. Few would debate the emotional overlay which is so common in almost every instance of asthma and practically every episode. Still, asthma is treated dramatically and potently with nebulizers and inhalers, pills and injections. Antibiotics as well as cortisone in one form or another are often part of the regimen. Breathing difficulties create large fears in patients, in families and in physicians, such that the Big Guns are often brought to bear on the problem at hand. This is very commonly the case even though mental-emotional components lie quite near the surface in almost all cases.

The next story illustrates how even from an early age, a child's emotions and will can have major effects on life and breath. I was doing Emergency Room duty at Irwin Army Hospital, Fort Riley, Kansas, one Sunday afternoon. Out of nowhere, a woman raced into the main treatment room with an infant in arms, yelling and screaming, "He's stopped breathing. He won't breathe. He's turning blue. Do something."

She left the child for the moment and ran away crying. The child was not quite blue. He must have had a breath or two when his mother wasn't looking. However, he wasn't breathing at the time.

I was out of my element as I was used to working with adults all the time. But, I got out my stethoscope and put it to his chest wondering how to proceed. As I did, the child took a big gulp, sputtered and coughed. He was back and breathing, sitting up and crying in a moment.

The boy's mother soon returned to give the rest of the story and say, "When he gets really angry, he stops breathing sometimes. He's done this before, but never for so long." Surely this mother and child, and many others in similar situations, needed more help than visits to the ER for urgent care.

This child's problem was much more dramatic and obvious than those of many asthmatics. But, emotional input is very important in most every incident. Asthma is clearly a dis-ease which requires much more than a stethoscope examination and pills for treatment.

- "Bladder infection" - This condition is so common and yet so matter-of-factly treated as purely physical - cranberry juice and medication - that the patient is given little of the real attention she needs. She - because this is far and away a more common female problem. UTI (urinary tract infection, again so-called) has many sexual and reproductive implications. Sexual history and candid conversation is key in most cases, but often not even considered. Tests (urinalysis, slides, cultures) and antibiotic treatment follow each other quickly. This dis-ease commonly overlaps with vaginitis which adds to clues of causation for those who have ears to hear.

There are many pathways to a "bladder infection." But, it is clear that most of the time these are not infections, but more irritation and congestion. A common variant is "honeymoon cystitis" which suggests overactivity being a cause. At the other end of the spectrum, these "infections" can appear when energy to the area is blocked or misdirected for one reason or another.

One case comes to mind with a young woman who had UTI symptoms and related a recent dream in which she was being chased by a man with a knife. Her symptoms were obviously influenced by thoughts and feelings regarding the threat of a knife (phallic symbol) and her need to be "chaste" rather than chased.

This woman hadn't even had sexual contact. Just the fears revealed by her dreams seemed enough for her to develop symptoms. Ah, but maybe there was more to the story than she told. We must consider the possible effect when layers - beyond the physical - of a person's being are involved.

- Fever - Fever is one of the most common symptoms to which people are prone. Unfortunately, patients and physicians often take a giant step to create a disease around it when fever lasts more than a few hours. All but low grade fever elicits treatment with aspirin, acetaminophen or the like.

Whether recognized or not, fever is often a sign of purification. The body takes on the job to clear, clean and change the interior milieu. To shift gears, to move to another level, to find a new point of balance. Adding medication to the mix often just makes more work for the system. Wise doctors and smart patients recognize that the body has its own wisdom and are prepared to give it time to "attend to business."

A Frugal Physician pays respect to the body as the instrument of a person's being and recognizes that there is a soul living through it. Each patient a physician meets has a different story which feeds into making that person a real person and weaves his/her unique drama of health and dis-ease.

Anything Can Cure Anything

Pondering again on Dr. Harper's unusual book title, we might take time to wonder if Anything Can Cure Anything. Why not?

Some sage proclaimed long ago, "One man's poison is another man's medicine." (A variation on the aphorism in Diagnosis . . .) The idea is still around and probably has some merit. It opens the field up for remedies of all sorts. A vast spectrum of therapies has been dispensed the world around over the ages, with still more continuing to appear. Like ground rhinoceros horns and mare's urine, animal organs, glands and gonads, strychnine and mercury compounds, apricot pits and asparagus ....

There surely is a connection between the proverb (above) and the following straightforward supposition: Many people are cured of illness - dis-ease - disease - even when the wrong or inadequate treatment is prescribed to them. Many more people recover with absolutely no treatment at all. Go figure.

I am reminded of when penicillin first appeared. It was such a wonderful drug that it "cured" in tiny doses. Manufacturing was limited and, at times, medics strained patient urine to recycle the penicillin. Was the drug really effective at such limited doses? How much of an effect did belief in a "promising" new ANTI-BIOTIC have then and now?

Let's brainstorm about how and why many people do so well in extreme conditions:

- Because they have lucky stars.
- Because stuff happens, good and bad.
- Because time takes care of most problems.
- Because dis-ease is self limiting.
- Because things usually work out for the best.
- Because the body heals itself.
- Because patients believe in their physicians.

Good work! They are probably all right. Let's start by considering the last reason. And touch on others here and there in subsequent chapters.

Dr. William Osler, in an article published in 1910 called The Faith that Heals, wrote, "Our results at the Johns Hopkins Hospital were most gratifying. Faith in Saint Johns Hopkins, as we called him, an atmosphere of optimism and cheerful nurses [notice Osler's hint as to the importance of *care*], worked just the same sort of cures as did Aesculapius at Epidaurus."

Osler was of the belief that most of the methods and treatments of his time were useless. (Things really haven't changed much from that angle.) He also remarked on repeated occasions that cures of major illnesses which he had overseen were due mostly to the patient's faith. "Far more important than what the physician does is the patient's belief in what the physician does." (*Aequanimitas*)

It seems that many Regular Physicians have forgotten or never understood Osler's simple observations. They really have deep and broad implications.

Norman Cousins tells (see Hospital Time) how he enlisted his primary physician's support - maybe even his enthusiasm - as Cousins took his unique route towards healing. The doctor's support was quite important to him. "Dr. Hitzig said it was clear to him that there was nothing undersized about my will to live. He said that what was most important was that I continue to believe in everything I had said. He shared my sense of excitement about the possibilities of my recovery and liked the idea of a partnership."

Faith can often trump science, or even common sense. Get a patient to believe in his/her doctor or treatment and more than half the battle is won. Putting it differently, I take the liberty of using a phrase brought home to me by my former wife, "It's not what you do, but how you do it."

The same method or remedy in one physician's hands may have entirely different results in another's. So, we now have a further very important variable in medicine and healing.

I am reminded of a brief conversation I had with a retired military patient at Martin Army Hospital in Fort Benning, Georgia.

That particular retiree seemed to spread his business between two states (Georgia and Alabama) as well as civilian and military facilities. He worked both sides to suit his desires and needs.

The retiree had some good things to say about the Army medical system. But, he couldn't restrain himself in praising his civilian general surgeon to the extent that, "I'd let him open my skull and cut on my brain if he thought it would help." Clearly, the man had faith in his MD. But, it may have been of the blind type which could lead both into a ditch.

As Dr. Osler earlier suggested the importance of patient over disease, he also exposed the practitioner factor. But the latter really turns back to a large degree on the patient. His or her belief system, sensitivity, receptivity, etc.

Some physicians have charisma. Some don't. They can substitute for that quality with compassion and concern, if they can draw that out from within themselves.

Patients respond to such qualities in those who "care" for them. Whether they consciously recognize the gifts of their care givers is irrelevant. The body and being are affected regardless.

People have been healing and being healed practically forever based on faith alone - or so it would seem. Regular Physicians believe that to be the case of the works of Chiropractors, Herbalists, Acupuncturists, Faith Healers, etc. They too often forget that faith has a lot to do with the effects of the pills they prescribe and the operations they perform.

More books can and should be written about the effects of faith in medical and healing processes. Faith is clearly of major importance. Yet, the system persists in spending huge monies on chemicals and devices to "fix the physical" with little awareness of the larger processes involved in healing.

Many things promote a sense of faith in a physician or other would-be healer:

Tradition	Mystique	Touch
Unique knowledge	Charisma	Power

The medical profession and its physicians possess most of these qualities, at least in potential. The MD degree carries with it a relatively monopolistic force, parochial knowledge, and a singular mystique. Power and authority have been vested in physicians by governments, courts, employers, schools, even churches. Little do the latter realize how little the former really know.

Yet, perception (faith, in other words) is a huge force. Even as the public whines about inadequate care, politicians ask for reform, and progressives want holistic practitioners, all of the above almost always turn back to orthodox MDs and the current system "when the chips are down." Stepping blatantly outside the controlling and politically invested medical box is rarely done. Alternative approaches for cancer and diabetes, etc. can bring lawsuits and other threats from the mainstream. The liberties and freedoms of life sometimes are cut short in the interests of disease care and medical orthodoxy. All this suggests that medicine is a truly powerful force to be reckoned with.

The Divine Right of Kings led to the tradition of "The Healing Touch" of monarchs in past ages. It is still in vogue in tribal societies and less developed regions of the world.

Sadly, touch is one of the least considered means by which medics can have dramatic effects on their patients. Touch is often taboo in the western world - "for safety's sake" - and even in the doctor's office - except in examination. How many patients simply need a hug and a good word to help them through?

I must tell a story which puts another slant on Hug Therapy. Years ago, I took myself to a week-long healing program in Virginia Beach, Virginia. Hugs were a common part of the experience and it seemed hugs might be another "treatment" I could share with my patients. I returned to the Troop Medical Clinic with the "hug bug." You know, hug therapy: "A hug a day."

I began dispensing hugs or at least pats on the shoulders to various and sundry patients. Private or sergeant, tall or short, robust or skinny, it didn't matter - at least for a while. The concept was great and is great, but the practice is not always so straightforward. "To hug or not to hug, that was the question." Not every situation or patient really called for a goodbye hug.

As part of my duties as Medical Consultant to the Alcohol and Drug Abuse Prevention and Control Program at Fort Riley, I interviewed each soldier who was enrolled - usually involuntarily - in that system. One particular female private who was abusing alcohol required two consultations for reasons which I don't recall.

At the end of our second meeting, I offered some words of counsel to the young woman and gave her a brief hug at the door. I thought nothing of the incident at the time. But, a week later the Division Surgeon called to report that the soldier had made accusations that I had tried to assault her in the office. The D.S. didn't even ask me about the episode, but merely told me of the allegation and of the other problems with which the woman was struggling at the time. Later on, I got a fuller report on her situation and was told that she had been acting out with alcohol as well as in other ways. I heard no more of the incident, but chastened myself about sharing hugs so freely. Sad to tell, "A hug a day is not always the best therapy."

In the West, Faith Healers have literally and metaphorically touched millions over the past 100+ years. From Holy Rollers and Pentecostals to more mainstream church men and women, healers have used the "power of the Holy Spirit" and unseen Presences, anointings and the group aura to change lives if not health of their followers. Without the simplest medical credentials, Aimee Semple McPherson, Oral Roberts, Kathryn Kuhlman, Ruth Carter Stapleton, Olga Worrall, Willard Fuller and others have lifted people out of their aches and pains for moments or for good, at little cost and to the betterment of "the whole family."

Historically, healers go much farther back than their medically trained descendants. The Christian Church has a long tradition of healing works from the time of the Essenes and of Jesus and his direct disciples into the creation of hospitals in the Middle Ages. Most modern hospitals were originally church owned and still have the aura of healing touch, however much it is fading now.

The concept of Placebo may be the most enlightening and bridging way to look at faith. Placebo has been studied medically ("further research is needed") and the idea garners interest as well as lip service if not wide acceptance among practitioners.

Placebo is simply an inert substance or inactive procedure which can be used in place of an "active" element to compare effects of the two in medical studies. Drug trials almost always include placebo (usually containing milk sugar) along with the medication being tested. Placebo invariably achieves positive response in 1/3 to 1/2 of patients.

In these trials, the difference in medication/s and placebo is intended to be the only variable. But, other unintended variables surely affect patients in their lives during drug trials.

While the "real drug" almost always beats placebo, one has to wonder how the sugar pill gets any positive results at all. Further, one wonders whether a little extra TLC shared with placebo users might be enough to cause the differences between drug and placebo effects to be neutralized. There are a host of other questions and implications with regard to placebos in drug trials and in use in medical practice.

The percentage of physicians who use placebos is almost beyond discovering. Guesstimates suggest placebo may be administered by 20 to 50 percent of physicians and 50 to 100 percent of nurses. The frequency of their use is totally unknown.

I remember requesting placebo (in little red capsules) to be stocked in Troop Medical Clinic #1, Fort Riley, Kansas. Lieutenant Colonel Davis, Division Surgeon, commented as he approved my request, "Do you have to tell patients you are giving them a placebo when you prescribe?"

I thought, "Duh!" when I read his response. "Why would I give a sugar pill to someone and tell him so?"

"Sergeant Patient, I'm writing you a prescription for a capsule which contains an inert substance. Theoretically, it should have absolutely no effect on you. But, I want you to give it a try, just the same. I guarantee it will work."

I probably used placebo in less than a handful of occasions during my medical career. I remember once prescribing for a young woman who was frequenting the Troop Medical Clinic with ever changing symptoms. She returned a few days after receiving an Obecalp (placebo spelled backwards) prescription, "Oh, those red capsules made me really sick. I can't take them, anymore."

I imagine that I was not particularly forceful in promoting the NEW medication with her. I certainly didn't believe in it very much. I had less experience with Placebo, than with many medications. I didn't have much faith in most of those, either.

There is so much evidence - not proof - that faith has truly major influences on patients, their care, and their prognosis in all sorts of situations. It behooves physicians and patients to pay heed.

The crux of the placebo-perception-faith situation seems to be the difference between just trying something and expecting it to work. The latter is much more likely to get a response. It has a good chance to work - at least for a while.

The Moral of this Story: Physicians need to have faith in their remedies. Patients even more so need faith in their physicians, Regular or Frugal or Otherwise. Faith is inexpensive, yet priceless.

Teaching and Learning

The importance of patients' faith in their physicians brings many intangibles - demeanor and attitudes, interests and aptitudes, hopes and aspiration - to the fore. Physicians are constantly expressing their talents and prejudices, ideals and struggles while they ply their trade and practice medicine.

Medicine surely has components of teaching and education, unconscious as well as conscious. The term DOCTOR comes from the Latin word for teacher. The best of doctors are teachers and practice following the premise: "Give a man a fish and you feed him for a day. Teach a man to fish and you feed him for a lifetime." Unfortunately, the present system makes it difficult to squeeze in teaching time during brief consultations.

So, much of teaching and learning happens unconsciously. This inner education cannot help but occur because physicians and patients, medical fixers and fixees have a great deal in common, more than you probably ever thought.

The vast majority of physicians are honestly and sincerely following their professions, seeking to aid and assist the patients who come to them. But in so doing, they are also learning about themselves through their patients.

Thus, they have conscious or unconscious need to deal with disease. They vicariously and at arms length - or greater, have the responsibility and opportunity to learn the lessons of their patients' problems. "Physician, heal thyself" ought to be part of medical training and creed. (See Patients of Job.)

Hard as it may be to believe, in many respects physician equates with patient. They really have much more in common than meets the eye. "A doctor who specializes in a disease is likely to fall victim to it, and this has always been understood in the medical profession. My old chief, a urologist, used to pray nightly, 'Oh, Lord, when Thou takest me, take me not through the bladder.' Cancer specialists are particularly apt to die of cancer and psychiatrists to commit suicide." (Margaret Millard)

A Real Physician is not just an attendant of the physical form, but a teacher in word, deed and presence to the minds and hearts and sometimes souls of his/her patients. When that is the case, true healing among patients - and providers - may be stimulated from time to time.

Whenever we are really about healing others, we are drawing forth (one definition of education) the best in them and reinforcing that in ourselves. The author, featuring himself to be a teacher, has had the chance to view and experience many varied teaching and learning opportunities in the course of 20 years passing through the medical profession. And many more in after years. Here are some which come to mind.

- First, I am reminded of my brother, the Salesman, who once said to the family minister, "You know, we are both in the sales business. I sell signs and you sell God."

The minister wasn't flattered, but certainly Brother had a point. We are all selling something; ourselves if naught else. Teaching and selling have a lot in common.

Physicians sell themselves as well as their products (pills and operations) and services (tests and procedures) and beliefs (based on medical knowledge). The better the physician's skills at teaching and selling, the better his patient is likely to respond.

- I remember meeting physicians whose name tags told reams about what they were teaching and learning - consciously or otherwise.

I was still a medical student when I got into conversation with a short brash, bulky, red-haired man in a business suit on a hospital elevator. He acted more like a salesman than a physician as he told stories and yucked it up. Actually, he was a surgeon.

Before his sales pitch was over and we got out of the elevator, he handed me his card which read Donald Butts, MD, Proctologist. I suspect he is still in practice and selling his service. I wonder what he is "up to now."

- Then, there was the cardiologist named Dr. Heart (maybe Hart). I didn't know him personally. I just heard bits of his story second hand. He must have needed more heart than some. His theme song could have been "You Gotta Have Heart."

You must have heard of Dr. Cutter. Of course, he was a general surgeon. And Dr. Blood, the hematologist. And Dr. Crabb who worked in oncology. (The crab is the astrological sign for Cancer and cancer itself is frequently called the "crab" in medical parlance.) How about Dr. Child, the pediatrician?

- Emma Jordan was a nurse practitioner with whom I worked at the A.R.E. Clinic. She was past 60 at the time. I can see her now. Thick hyperopic glasses, permed and dyed short gray hair, a lilt to her voice and an often seeming frustrated air. She waddled a bit like she had arthritis. It can be hard to get old even for a medical person.

Emma had the consolation of working with patients who were a lot like her. Or certainly became that way by the time they had been on her panel for a while.

Emma was obviously post-menopausal and on hormones. So were a swath of her patients. She was hypothyroid and taking some form of thyroxin. As were many of her patients.

Emma regularly set up patients for glucose tolerance tests looking for hypoglycemia which she had. There were a few other recurring ailments like sinusitis and candidiasis which were common to herself and patients. Emma had companions on the way with her dis-ease, as she undoubtedly saw herself in many of her patients. Like attracts like, which certainly creates learning opportunities.

- Medicine has other ways of teaching, some very mystical and removed from regular eyes and common thinking. Nonetheless, mythic guardians such as Asclepius and Chiron must watch over the comings and goings of its practitioners. They looked after me.

You say, "I don't believe in that! You're pulling my leg." Not so. Let me give you something we might both agree on which may also cause you to rethink your disbelief in medical guardians.

You must have driven in heavy big city highway traffic and wondered more than a few times, "How can this crowd of lethal vehicles charging around at high rates of speed keep from regular mishaps, injuries and fatalities? With all these oblivious drivers, texting, phoning, lunching, radio listening and map reading, how do people keep from harming each other every day?"

Well, my answer is "Surely, there are invisible Lords of Traffic which keep us safe most of the time. When our number is up, They keep those whose numbers aren't out of our way. Think about it!"

Similarly, there must be Angels - Spirits - Guardians who watch over us in our health and in our disease. They only permit that which is our due to come to us. Since "as we sow, so shall we reap," we must also be kept from reaping what we have not sown.

Asclepius is the patron of healing who carries medics through the trials and tribulations of the profession and guides them according to their effort and motive. Chiron has the special task of coming sooner or later to every physician to teach him/her about mortality, pain, and humanity. Personally and not just in the guise of his/her patients.

Chiron is the sign of the healer and wounded one. Like Gus Wood (see below), we all have wounds and weaknesses. Until physicians grapple with them and learn from them, their abilities to aid and heal others are surely limited. The lessons of Chiron some day will return intentionally to the medical curriculum as they were centuries ago. (See Patients of Job.)

- All of us, including physicians, are constantly drawing the experiences we need to enrich our path through life. We thus meet ourselves coming and going. MEETING SELF is our major course of study. Eventually - it may take a very long time - we learn the course of instruction ordained for us.

One needy learner in my Family Practice residency was Dr. Gus Wood. Gus was "a hell of a guy," but had a "hell of a problem," as well. Practically everyone smiled at and bantered with Gus, listening to him and his stories. Everyone was glad he was in the program and in the hospital.

But, Gus wasn't so sure about being there. Gus wasn't sure about most anything. He lacked self-confidence and self-esteem. He was always telling or demonstrating his weaknesses to staff and fellow residents alike. Maybe to his patients as well.

Wood was tall - well over six feet - and stocky. He filled out his uniform so he looked the part of an aging military officer. Gus had a large round face, lined forehead, and a scalp that was bald except for a few wisps over the ears and around the back. Tiny bubbles of sweat often oozed out his pores. Gus always has a hanky handy to absorb trickles of errant perspiration.

His big face generally wore a broad grin - except when it didn't. Like when he was worried or fretting over something or someone. Gus was the Teddy Bear of the resident bunch. He had a heart of gold and was truly concerned about his patients. He worried about them and cried over them when they hurt or died. He cried on other occasions.

Dr. Wood was the oldest resident in the program. He was in his forties while the rest of us were still in our twenties. Gus had been practicing medicine here and there within the military and other federal agencies for many years. Gus had traveled the world far and wide looking for fulfillment and for himself. He had drunk heavily at times along the way and "taken the cure." He had long abused his body, but at the time limited his vices to chain smoking and coffee guzzling. Altogether, the years told on him.

On occasion, fellow residents would drop in on Gus when he was on call and staying in the doctor's quarters. If we found him stretched out with his shoes off, we would be overwhelmed by the pungent and fetid aroma emanating from his feet. No amount of foot powder or Odor Eaters could ever neutralize the fumes and miasms which radiated from the soles of his poor feet. Gus's feet became the center of puns and jokes, smirks and smiles. We all knew that we were in imminent olfactory danger when we found Gus crashed in the call room. Regardless, we all thought Gus was great and would never avoid a chance to spend a moment with him.

Gus suffered not just over patients, but also over himself. Working in the government service since medical school, Dr. Wood had neglected to take a medical board exam and was therefore unlicensed to practice in any state. He was not legitimized to do a civilian practice and he didn't plan to stay in the military forever.

So, Gus forced himself to go back into formal training and brush up for medical boards. He joined us as a second-year family practice resident. But, Wood was forever carrying his perceived lack of knowledge and obvious lack of confidence almost literally on his sleeve. I can see him now shuffling down the hospital hallway, worrying about something and looking for a colleague to lean on. He usually had his hands full of charts and papers. The pockets of his long white coat overflowed with notebooks and cheat sheets, pens and pencils, instruments and dosage calculators.

At one time, I suggested that we sew a large pocket on the back of his medical coat so that he might carry for "easy reference" a copy of Harrison's thousand-page, ten-pound *Principles of Internal Medicine*. The funny thing was that if such a pocket had been feasible, Gus would have sewn it himself. It might have eased a bit of his anxiety about not knowing enough.

How much was enough? Gus didn't know. He just had the ever-present sense of inadequacy and continued to tell anyone who would listen how much he didn't know. Eventually, the residency staff heard his refrain one time too many. At the end of the year, they told Gus, "We've decided you don't know enough medicine, Dr. Wood, to be advanced in the program. You also lack sufficient confidence in the abilities you do have. You must repeat the second year of the training."

Gus's two-year residency turned into a three-year program. I suppose that he was ultimately relieved when the decision was made. I assume that somehow the extra year made some difference. For, Gus completed the program. The last I heard from him, he was practicing at Fort Polk, Louisiana, and preparing anxiously to take the medical licensing exam in Texas.

We all learn the hard way, at least in some areas of our life. No one has a "free ride." If Gus had perceived himself as we did him, his battle would have been greatly eased. He already had qualities of heart and compassion that some physicians never get close to.

Instead of carrying a medical textbook on his back, he actually carried an invisible shining heart which touched many people. That is a gift which a Frugal Physician gradually develops and shares quite freely.

- Another physician named George Hart (not related to the cardiologist) comes to mind. When I first met Dr. Hart, he was working as a psychiatrist at the Yellowstone Boys and Girls Ranch west of Billings, Montana. We sat across from each other for lunch at a downtown cafe with a mutual friend in between. George's story or parts of it - unfolded quickly. He was obviously a sensitive and caring medical professional. A soft-spoken, graying man in his early 60s, Hart had recently moved his second family to the West.

As opposed to many psychiatrists who seem to hide behind desks and beards and pipes, George was more than willing to share his story and expose himself. The most poignant part of his life up to the present time concerned an experiment in the 60s and 70s when he purchased Great Duck Island (off the coast of Maine) to treat and nurture psychotic patients without drugs.

He apparently had some successes, but he also took on a large burden which modern psychiatry pretty much avoids by prescribing high powered drugs to sedate and pacify difficult patients. That was the tipping point. He helped others, but to his own detriment.

In the midst of his storytelling, George recalled the beauty of the island and the variety of animals which roamed its open spaces. Then, he got absorbed in remembering a striking experience. He was alone walking the land in a pensive state. He turned down a path and encountered a lone DEER. He stood within feet of it. Their eyes met and George had some sort of ecstatic moment of other-worldly communication. This caused him to sob openly in the midst of lunch. Which was fine with me, but may have startled our mutual friend who was a rather interiorized computer geek.

This encounter was obviously a profoundly affecting experience for him, though he didn't seem to recognize it as such. I spent occasional moments with George in coming weeks and months and, on occasion, sought to get him to revisit the DEER meeting and draw out more meaning from it.

To do so became a more incumbent proposition when I met his new family and visited their rural property in the direction of Red Lodge Mountain. Dr. Hart had a young wife, Martha, and two little children, a boy and a girl. George seemed to have found family success later in life as well as a nurturing retreat in the Montana countryside.

When he was not occupied with his professional work at the Boys and Girls Ranch, he could relax and enjoy his own ranch. The ranch had no cows or pigs or sheep or even horses, but it did have dozens of DEER.

That seemed to be a perfectly poetic sequel to the Duck Island story. Martha spoke of George going out to spend time with the deer in the evening. Sometimes, he took a portable radio and tuned in classical music for them.

There was a flip side to the idyllic picture, though. Mrs. Hart told how difficult it was for George to do veterinary tasks with the animals. Vaccination, tagging, de-horning and minor surgeries on them created pains as well as chores for him. He seemed to feel what his animals felt.

What was even more disturbing for George was his intention to eventually slaughter the animals and sell their meat to area restaurants. But, he didn't seem to be fully aware of the conflict. He was an extraordinarily sensitive helping person who worked with disturbed youth and cared for some of God's equally sensitive creatures. Deer are gentle, inquisitive, and acute creatures. Simply put DEER are DEAR.

They are much like George was.

On more than one occasion, I tried to suggest that there might be an alternative to slaughtering the animals. "If these deer can nurture and heal you, maybe they can do the same for young people like those who are struggling at the Boys and Girls Ranch."

The idea seemed to go nowhere. George thought his ranch had to pay like similar operations. Although I don't think George got very far along in his plan to make his ranch venison available to local eateries. Life has a way of getting in the way of plans.

One day out of the blue, Bill, our mutual friend, told me, "George is in rehab at St. Vincent's Hospital." I went up to see him. It was never quite clear whether he had had a stroke or a heart attack. George was a psychiatrist, not an internist. Still, the episode gave him a jolt and laid him up in the hospital for quite a period.

He recovered and was able to return to work at the Boys and Girls Ranch. He later told me that it was in this time period that he had an epiphany of sorts. It came to him that he had been dealing with Attention Deficit Disorder his whole life without realizing it. And he needed to do something about it.

The obvious question seemed to be how was a man with ADD ever able to get through college, medical school, residency. This psychiatrist, past 60 years of age, decided after all those years that he had his own mental problems. George determined that he needed to do something about them. And he did. He convinced the family practice doctor at the Ranch to prescribe Ritalin for him.

George was lost from sight for some time. I eventually heard he was living at the Sage Apartments in Billings. I went for a visit and found him holed up in a dinky flat. His place was cluttered and in disarray. His mattress was spread on the floor without frame or accessories. He made no apologies but was glad for the visit. Then, he recited the update of his life since our last meeting.

It seems Ritalin pushed George over the edge and into a nervous breakdown. His psychosis had played out in full view of his wife and children. Mrs. Hart initiated divorce proceedings after George Hart was sent as a patient to the State Hospital in Warm Springs. He eventually was released and returned to what appeared to be a totally empty life.

I don't know the final chapters of George's story. I discovered that he died in 1997 (I last saw him in 1993) in Butte as noted in a small obituary in a Harvard University bulletin.

At least two recurring thoughts come to my mind when George Hart appears there. One concerns whether or not Dr. Hart had Attention Deficit Disorder. That was his belief and caused him to act accordingly at a critical passage. Then, Life really got his Attention and he had the rest of his few years to consider the consequences.

More benevolently, I have always wondered whether George had the capacity to learn the lesson of his meeting with the deer on Duck Island. If there was a lesson? Had he learned it, could his life have ended differently?

The DEER definitely got his attention in that poignant moment. Could he have retrieved its essence? Or, was he fated to end his days so sadly? I wish to think that George had the potential to recognize himself in that lone, lovely DEER who looked deeply into his being. George might have made a large step by merely realizing that from ancient times a DEER has been known also as a HART.

- One of the major lessons of medicine as well as life is suggested in the Golden Rule which is part of practically every religious tradition on Earth. "Do unto others."

Unfortunately, religion and spirituality aren't part of the medical curriculum. Like so many other key aspects of practically every person's (and patient's) life. A Frugal Physician has so many of the deepest and most important things to learn after s/he leaves the corridors of his/her medical school.

"Love your neighbor (patient), as your self." But, how often is the cart put before the horse? Physicians are constantly about the work of helping, repairing, fixing others. Or intending so.

How can a physician truly love-help-aid-heal a patient until s/he has developed the love of self? Self respect, esteem and love must arise within a doctor, or s/he is just a technician. And not necessarily a useful one.

We all must develop self love. So that we have some real love to give away. Whether that is in the context of business or office, home or neighborhood. The physician is not alone in this part of life. But has a special calling to find the key to open the heart.

You wonder: "A doctor is supposed to keep a distance from his patients. Be a professional and do his job. Now, you say he is supposed to be spending more time loving him/her self and others than addressing his/her occupation?"

Maybe the quickest way to answer that one is to point out the obvious fact that many, many people find their way to the doctor's office because they are in need of attention, reassurance, some form of love. The shortest route to addressing those patients' problems is to listen to them and to BE with them.

It seems more than likely that the vast majority of clinic patients would do better with a listening ear than another prescription. For many people, a trip to see the doctor at the clinic is a way to experience more than the four walls and the television, to get out of the house, to have company and conversation.

- A next step in medical practice will then be such that patients become brothers, family, parts of the self. Doctor and patient, patient and doctor are really no different.

Standing face to face, the patient should be a mirror for the physician. The patient is most truly part of the physician's larger self. He or she only appears to be separate from the physician. Appearances can be deceiving, as we well know.

I assume that it is still common for patients to be treated as less than - needy, sick, helpless, etc. Even difficult patients deserve more than being called names which place them in Outer Darkness.

Health care providers must learn to do unto others (their patients) as they would do unto themselves. "As ye do unto the least of these..."

- The practice of medicine and the life of patients is often of one of "hurry up and wait." Patients can handle that. They have no choice. But, physicians don't manage well under that scheme of things. They like to be in control and make things happen. "It needs to be done and as soon as possible."

Ah but, "Rome wasn't built in a day," and neither was the patient's body nor the practitioner's. Patients need patience and so do physicians. Patience is a great virtue and worthy of efforts to bring it into a physician's armamentarium. "In patience, possess ye your souls." (Saint Luke)

Time is one of the great healers. One that comes to the aid of doctors more often than they realize. They might endeavor to use it more consciously.

How long did it take to make a human being or a body part the first time around? How long did it take for the patient to get into his/her condition? Is it reasonable to expect that illness and injury should be reversed more quickly than it took for them to develop and create symptoms?

There is much for all of us to experience and learn. Hopefully, we can teach and learn more gently and kindly from each other in the coming times.

Lip Service

A few generations ago, going into medicine, nursing and ancillary professions often required many years of real sacrifice. These were truly service careers. Physicians were paid sparingly if at all in training and earned little in the early years of practice. Medical men had to fight for specialized training, take what they could get, and work like the dickens. They were sure to be in debt for many years while getting their practices started and established. Big houses and long vacations often didn't occur until late in careers. Physicians may not have been necessarily frugal in those days, but they certainly didn't get well-heeled in a hurry.

Financial rewards have changed dramatically from era to era. Sacrifice is hardly an apt word in recent times. Physicians are handsomely paid from the get-go. Salaries start in the six figures range.

Registered nurses and even CNAs garner substantial wages.

In the "olden days," hospital workers barely made ends meet. I remember my maiden Aunt Elizabeth, a registered nurse for fifty years, bemoaning the long hours and low pay she accepted while working on hospital wards. I also recall her pulling out one of the many scraps which she kept in one drawer or another. A little article detailed the duties of a floor nurse in an era just before hers. "The Frugal Nurse" might have been a fitting title for that period. Among other parsimonious tasks, the nurse in training was directed to conserve her one pencil until it was little more than a nub.

Service like frugality has gone by the wayside to a large degree in medical practice and many other areas of daily life. (Consider for a moment the United States Postal Service. It seems that Americans got more SERVICE when it was the Post Office than since it became the USPS.) These days, it is the physician's schedule, plan and protocol that are most important. The patients' needs often rank second or further down the order. The reader undoubtedly has stories which support this observation.

Real service puts the customer-patient first when at all possible. It also points to the importance of care and compassion in medical practice. How often have you felt that you were really the most important person in your physician's day - if only for a moment? How do you rate your physician's bedside manner? Is s/he really with you - present - when entering the room? Or just running from one obligation to another?

Compassion doesn't cost a penny, but it can be invaluable. It can be as simple as taking one extra moment to show care and concern. I saw this demonstrated ONCE in medical school during my third year while I was on Dr. Red Duke's Surgery Service. Duke was a hard-charging, no-nonsense cowboy who was also Director of the Hermann Hospital Emergency Center at the time. He eventually became famous by doing a syndicated *Health Reports* TV show and by having his life portrayed by Dennis Weaver as *Buck James* also on television.

The wiry, redheaded, bespectacled Duke would careen through Hermann Hospital corridors with our entourage keeping close pace behind him. He was quick to make decisions and move on to the next task. But . . .

But, he wasn't shy about spending time and getting close to patients, an unusual occurrence it seemed, especially for a surgeon. I remember our group standing behind him during morning rounds in a man's hospital room as Duke traded questions and answers back and forth with his patient. Something caught his attention and caused him to move closer to the man's bed. Then, he sat down on the edge. He motioned for us to leave the room as I heard him say to our patient, "Have you got time to talk?"

"Have you got time to talk?" Consider the implications of that remark made by a busy surgeon to a patient lying in a hospital bed.

Communication is so important in the present age that it is hard to imagine life without mouths flapping and words flowing from them. Yet, there must be times when we all wonder if our wind is worth the effort, especially when we remember it takes two to have a conversation.

Medical practitioners use clever and honed questioning in their desire to quickly get to "the bottom of the case." However, these rote litanies often elicit flat, dull or meager responses. This causes physicians to find what they are looking for. But, will the result be good for their customers: patients with unique and personal problems?

As a medical student, I was at times intimidated by surgeons. They were larger than life in some respects. And they seemed to like it that way. "We're saving lives every day." Especially trauma surgeons, like Dr. Duke.

Blood and guts never suited me much, even though I entered medical school thinking I wanted to become an emergency room physician. Having spent a tour as a corpsman in Vietnam and worked in three other ERs before med school, I had been excited by the speed and drama of the Emergency Room. Patching people up and putting them back together seemed a magical calling. But, many things are not just as they appear to be.

Neither was Dr. Duke. He had that brash "cut him open and stop the bleeding" part to him. But, he also was a wise ol' country boy. I suspect he had more than a little common sense and compassion in him. He was an enthusiastic cheerleader for his brand of medicine, for his trauma center, and for the medical school. He no doubt cheered for patients, too.

Enough to take time out from playing Chief of the Surgical Team to close the door and sit and converse with another soul. "I wish I could have been a fly on the wall of that hospital room," as my mother might have said. I might have learned even more. Of course, Duke might have just wanted to have a man-to-man conversation about the Texas Longhorns' coming season. But, I have to believe he had more than football on his mind.

Healing comes in many forms and I am quite sure that Red Duke knew it. If a man needed the knife, so be it. If he needed some one to talk to and hear "the rest of the story," Dr. Duke could surely handle that.

That episode stuck in my mind, like many others. I carried it with me until many years later after I had "taken down my shingle." I was sitting close to another man's bedside in a hospital room in Montana. I had shied away from medicine and hospitals for quite a few years when I "fell into" a job in the education department of Billings Deaconess Hospital. Drawing on my medical experience and computer interests, I did program development for hospital health and safety training.

During that time, I got it into my head to do some volunteer work on the wards. When asked how I would like to help, I said, "I would like to read to patients."

For other volunteers that usually meant newspapers, but I wanted to read books. I did so with just three or four patients. But, one patient made it all worth the while and kept me reading with him for some months.

Mr. Les Trafton had been in the hospital for many weeks by the time I arrived on the scene. A retirement-age man, Les had lung cancer which prompted removal of one lung. He arrested on the operating table and a series of sad complications ensued.

Trafton had a tracheotomy and could not talk, but was clearly pleased to have new and regular company. His wife, Max, and sister-in-law were often in attendance when I appeared several times a week to read Louis L'Amour books to Les. We went through a number of L'Amour westerns, then a modern novel, *Last of the Breed*. I eventually got my fill of western novels and the Sackett family by the time months later when Les was finally transferred for to his hometown hospital in Miles City.

Along the way, I became part of the family, so to speak. I'm sure Les appreciated the male attention, but the two ladies did so as well. In future months, I made two visits to the Traftons at their home. Hospitality replaced hospital time.

I could only take so much Louis L'Amour and got agreement for me to read another classic western, *Shane*. Just before the Traftons left town, Max and I went out and rented the video. The three of us watched the movie version of *Shane* in one sitting and drew even closer together.

I can't help recalling moments when Trafton's thoracic surgeon "peeked his head" into the room or stood at the foot of the bed and made his daily hospital call. In later weeks, Les's tracheotomy had been repaired and he was able to speak. Still, the give and take between physician and patient seemed miniscule and distant. I wonder if Les's surgeon ever sat at the edge of his bed and had a man-to-man, heart-to-heart talk with him. I wonder if the surgeon ever did that with any patient. Did he ever take time to read a western to anyone?

Many people wish that old-time country doctors were still in business. The search may not be in vain when there are old-time country patients on the lookout for that supposedly dying breed.

Hard-charging Dr. Red Duke took time to sit on the edge of his patient's bed to visit with him. To be a friend as well as a physician. Both men undoubtedly gained something from the spontaneous exchange. There seem to be many reasons to believe that more physicians, frugal and otherwise, can do much the same.

Buddha Ears

Dr. Jim Duke knew how to open the door for patients to tell their stories. I never had that "fly on the wall experience with him." So, it's hard to even guess what kind of conversation and stories he may have elicited.

I do know, however, that another physician with whom I worked was told all manner of tales. She seemed to attract and collect them. Eventually, she authored a book or two calling on her gifts of a listening ear and warm heart.

Gladys McGarey co-founded (with her husband) the A.R.E. Clinic in the 70s as an effort to promote the holistic principles of Edgar Cayce, the Sleeping Prophet. The Clinic became a training ground for many physicians, like myself, and other medical care professionals who passed momentarily through its doors. I often thought that the McGareys had, consciously or unconsciously, tried to recreate the halcyon influences of ancient Egypt. What better place than Phoenix, Arizona?

The best parts of the Clinic were manifested in its one and two-week residential programs. The former was called Creative Living and the latter The Temple Beautiful.

Drs. Gladys and Bill were pioneering when they started the A.R.E. Clinic. They also helped create similar organizations, such as the American Holistic Medical Association. Gladys has been called the "Mother of Holistic Medicine."

Bill was a Scorpio and acted as the Head of the A.R.E. Clinic. Gladys, a Sagittarian, was clearly the Heart. I first spent time with them on a one-month Family Practice elective in my senior year of medical school. It was another learning get-away from the Texas Medical Center.

By the time I left the US Army Medical Corps in 1981, the Clinic seemed the obvious next step on my career and life path. Also by that time, Gladys had a bigger day-to-day role in the Clinic as Bill took on more administrative, fundraising, and writing work. So, I saw a lot more of Gladys than Bill which was fine with me.

Gladys was then approaching 60 and gray around the gills, if not more. But, she aged radiantly then and probably now as she has passed 90 and still practices medicine. There were a number of remarkable things about Gladys. She stood out in any group.

Gladys was a real inspiration to most everyone who met her whether or not they agreed with her brands of medicine and/or spirituality. She greeted physicians, patients, and public in the same attentive, present, softly beaming manner. She always wore colorful clothes which were usually accented with Southwest Indian designs, alternatively East Asian patterns. Silver and turquoise invariably hung from her ears and around her neck. The white medical coat, often obligatory, added to the aura.

One picture sticks in my mind of her wearing her favorite dangling jewelry which became commingled - then tangled - with her stethoscope and tethered eyeglasses. Then, she had a devil of a time unraveling the mess.

To add to the image, Gladys was fairly tall. Her longish hair was often rolled into a bun and secured to the top of her head making Gladys look Buddha-esque. Her ear lobes seemed as long as the Buddha's, and not just because of the presence of earrings. The Orient was written all over her.

I can see her now. Her aging mystical eyes gently peering into and through the people who approached her asking for advice and attention. I suspect she was not only looking into others but into herself all at the same time. The dreamy, intuitive Gladys was no scientist, though she would like to have been. Dr. Gladys was a feeler and a healer - a woman with a big heart and a physician with charisma.

She told her own stories of growing up in India with parents who were osteopathic physicians and missionaries, but not necessarily in that order. When the old adage of "You are what you eat," was once spoken, she had to add, "and what you think about what you eat." Gladys recalled that the missionary life in India kept her family close to the poverty line. They often had little to eat. "So, we prayed over it. And I'm sure the prayers made a difference."

Gladys also told stories of her memories of India in more distant times. She remembered being midwife for Mumtaz Mahal (1593-1630), the wife of Shah Jehan who was a great Mogul Emperor. Mumtaz Mahal ("beloved ornament of the palace") died while bearing the 14th child for her emperor husband. Shah Jehan was so bereft by the loss that he built the Taj Mahal in her memory.

In this life, Gladys started as a mother of five, later graduated from medical school and became a family practitioner. Her main interests were quite naturally women and children.

That work was the source for many of her stories and more than a few heartaches, because she cared so much for her patients. While her husband drifted away from Gladys as well as from caring for patients, she has stayed with direct care for over 50 years.

One of her tales sticks in my mind. Probably because I had a patient during my brief A.R.E. Clinic stint who had a lot in common with her own. The story concerned a young woman who came to see Gladys for a rash over the course of some weeks. She complained of a reddened, itchy area in between her breasts which wouldn't go away regardless of treatment.

On a return visit, Gladys peered more deeply and asked the patient to do the same. She seemed to see a pattern which the skin condition made on her patient's chest. "I wonder if maybe your rash is trying to tell you something." Dr. Gladys stood the woman in front of a mirror and asked her to stare at her uncovered torso.

Embarrassed and scared, the woman said, "I'm sorry. I don't see anything. Maybe I'm dense."

Then, Gladys suggested that the patient use her imagination and turn the rash upside down. "That's pretty strange. Why, it almost looks like an A."

Dr. Gladys then proceeded to tell her the story of *The Scarlet Letter* made famous in Nathaniel Hawthorne's book. The main character, Hester Prynne, always wore a scarlet cloth in the shape of the letter A over her outer garment after she was exposed as an Adulteress by the elders of her Puritan Boston community.

That story opened the gates for the patient to break down, cry and tell her own tale. Gladys suggested that she had unconsciously created her own mark as a result of her self condemnation. She somaticized (embodied) her guilt over an adulterous affair. But, she was the only one who could ever read the branding because of its inverted position.

There are so many dimensions to our lives, our illnesses and our healings. Most physicians and patients miss all but the superficial ones, those being the most obvious. Sometimes, they even escape their detection.

During my brief tenure at the A.R.E. Clinic, I cared for a patient named Marjorie Barker. To this day, I don't recognize the full implications of my care for Mrs. B. You see, while I attended the retirement-aged patient with metastatic breast cancer, my mother was (in her 70s) in the midst of her own struggle with the same sort of disease. I might well have been treating my own mother in the guise of Marjorie Barker.

I shall not forget the moment I first faced Mrs. B. To understate things, our meeting was more than a bit of a shock to me. I walked nonchalantly into the treatment room with a new patient chart which simply stated, "Fluid on patient's abdomen." I stood in front of a forlorn and frightened woman who was uncomfortably seated on the treatment table. Her story - at least the surface of it - was quickly understood. Mrs. Barker's body was filled with fluid from her diaphragm down. Her belly was bulging and her legs were thick as logs. But, her arms were skinny and her face was thin and drawn as to make her look almost emaciated.

Marjorie's cancer had spread into her abdomen, her lymphatic system was blocked with tumor, and her belly was filled with water. Mrs. B. merely wanted the fluid tapped so that she could rest comfortably. Sadly, she related the story of her previous visit to Doctor's Hospital where the fluid had last been drained off. According to her words, she had been mistreated by the physician who had performed the procedure. He had badgered her about getting more chemotherapy and having drugs instilled into her belly to slow the cancer's effects. The doctor bad-mouthed Marjorie when she said she wasn't interested in more therapy. With a stifled sob, Mrs. B. told me, "I have enough to deal with without fighting a nasty doctor. You won't do that to me, will you?"

I agreed to work with Mrs. Barker in a way that fit her needs and wishes. We made an appointment to perform the procedure the next afternoon when a drainage set could be procured. That day, with some trepidation, I performed my first paracentesis. Well over a gallon of pale yellow fluid poured from Mrs. B.'s swollen middle. Her ballooned appearance quickly changed. Marjorie was greatly relieved and equally appreciative.

Thereafter, we repeated the process every four or five days. As time went on, Marjorie caught on that the Clinic care was quite unlike her Doctor's Hospital experience. She also gathered that I was of a much different breed than the last physician she had encountered. Mrs. B. eventually agreed to our starting some Cayce-type therapies along with her regular abdominal taps. As we initiated the new remedies, I began to get a sense of Marjorie's life and struggles.

I gave her some dietary suggestions and recommended the use of castor oil packs at home. The most curious treatment we offered her involved ultraviolet light. Actually, it was the most exotic modality I ever "experimented" with in my medical career. After Marjorie swallowed a capsule of Animated Ash in water and waited thirty minutes for the substance to begin circulating in her blood stream, we shined an ultraviolet light through a green glass filter onto her chest for a few short minutes. According to the Cayce readings, the light treatment focalized the animated ash and liberated healing ozone in her affected tissues.

Whether it really worked in such a manner is only speculation, but Marjorie began to improve dramatically. Her weight increased, the tumorous discoloration of her skin began to coalesce and shrink, her need for fluid taps decreased in frequency, and her attitude was more buoyant and hopeful.

The "effect" of Mrs. B.'s tumor on her skin was something totally new to me. All over her left chest where her breast had been removed was a great dry, reddish-purple blotch. It startled everyone who ever helped with Mrs. B.'s treatment. I imagine that it was equally unnerving to Marjorie as well.

The more treatments we did with Marjorie, the more it became apparent that her discolored chest had its own story to tell. It seemed that "Adultery" was a hidden concern to her. Middle-aged Marjorie had been "living in sin" for years. She had a grown family and mother living nearby who helped her during the time of her illness. I had no sense of them ever accusing her. Marjorie's "Arrangement" was actually a common-day relationship of convenience. Ostensibly, Marjorie did not marry her live-in because of financial reasons. Should she have taken a second spouse her income would have been greatly reduced.

As Mrs. B. improved, I tiptoed around trying to get her some supportive counseling. I sensed that if I was too direct with her, she would run away. I suggested that she do some biofeedback and guided imagery work. She agreed to "think about it." And, she continued to "think about it" as long as I saw her. In her latter visits, Marjorie remarked that her live-in had been telling neighbors that her condition was worsening. That behavior obviously hurt her, especially since she was actually much improved at the time.

At our last meeting, she announced her crosstown move to stay with her mother. She apparently left her man without a word. On the whole, the decision seemed appropriate and good. Strikingly, Mrs. Barker made another choice at the same time - to discontinue her Clinic visits and abdominal taps. The decision was not spoken directly to me. It only became apparent through her mother's communications and her failure to return to see me.

Marjorie died a short time after her last trip to the Clinic. At first, I felt that maybe we had wasted her time and put her through needless procedures by treating her. Maybe I was no better than the physician she encountered at Doctor's Hospital weeks before. Ultimately, I rationalized that we had done the best we knew how. We treated Margaret like a human being and gave her respect. We also gave her a ray of hope which may have lasted long enough for her to make some small but critical decisions in her final days.

There is a short postscript to her story. At the 1982 A.R.E. Clinic Symposium, I made a presentation about my work with Marjorie. Mrs.

B. was in the midst of her "remission" at the time, but she understandably chose not to attend the meeting. The morning of the talks, I waited my turn to speak while seated in the midst of a crowd of four or five hundred. I felt relatively well-prepared for the few moments I was to have at the microphone. But, the longer I sat waiting to "go on," the more nervous I became. My heart began to thump in my chest and my whole body seemed to buzz. I tried to center myself, relax, meditate - but to no avail.

Mercifully, my turn arrived and I said my piece. The words came out although my mouth was dry as cotton. I knew I was quivering in my shoes, but I hoped no one in the audience noticed. It was probably hard to miss my stage anxiety, but I received only compliments after completing my presentation. Nobody mentioned my "nerves," that day.

However back at the Clinic a few days later, I ran into Dr. Bill. He started talking about the symposium and threaded his way into a tale about his graduation day at medical school. Bill recounted how he was to have given the valedictory speech before his graduating class. But, he became so petrified that he couldn't even mount the speaker's platform and left the convocation in keen embarrassment. Bill looked right through me and said, "I was paying attention during your case presentation the other day. If someone had asked me, I would have said, 'You were scared spitless.'" I laughed. We both laughed. He told me there was hope. He was right.

Well, it's all practice. Medical or otherwise. And, everybody has a story. Probably many stories which make up the bigger one. Dr. Gladys helped teach me that. As she has undoubtedly done for many others.

Illness and dis-ease are always part of larger scenarios. Wise Physicians, like Gladys McGarey, take the time to make listening to life episodes and stories key to their medical work.

Good Hands

It has seemed to me for the longest time that the use of the hands - the sense and gift of touch - is probably the most underused element in medicine and in life. We touch our pets more than we do our children and mates. We spend more time polishing the floor or waxing the car than we would ever imagine caressing our family members. Pressing the flesh, a peck on the cheek or a quick hug is about as touchy-feely as we westerners are bold enough to be with neighbors and kin.

"Got to keep our distance." "Don't get too close." "Careful about other people's boundaries." "Don't be invading someone else's space." We project these thoughts and words onto others largely out of our own fears and discomforts with regard to touch and proximity to others.

Regardless of where this modern thinking begins, it carries over into medical practice. As stated earlier, medics rarely touch their patients except for physical exams or doing one sort of procedure or another, often invasive. And these are always done wearing plastic gloves. Sterility and safety, caution and precaution clearly overrule care and compassion.

Some of our modern ways might make one wonder how humans ever reached the 21st century, especially in such numbers. Danger and disease, germs and microbes, not to mention wars and violence have been with us practically forever, it seems. How did we manage without sterility and masks and gloves, quarantines and isolation procedures, protective webs and guards of so many kinds?

The writer thinks the benefits of all such methods have been vastly overrated and magnified beyond the realms of good sense. They have been good for many medical businesses - the makers of gloves, Lysol, Betadine, and sterilizing agents and equipment. But, not for human beings and the contact and communication they need and often crave.

Fortunately on the fringes of medicine lie small islands of workers who express sanity and humanity, and give the simple offering of touch to aid the ill and injured - WITHOUT GLOVES. Massage therapists, energy workers, and hands-on healers fill a huge gap in the medical system. They do such for a relative few, in part, because most of them work outside the medical and insurance systems which control and monopolize medical monies.

The medical system itself relies largely on physical therapists who until recently touched their patients little more than their physician referrers. Fortunately, PTs have begun to hear about the benefits of touch gained by patients who have gone outside the system, paid out of their pockets, and experienced things that medics have shunned for decades if not centuries.

The power and influence of touch have been known for ages. Yet with touch being hard to test and quantify, book-based physicians have deemed it unscientific. Relatively recent inroads have been made into the system as osteopathy (now osteopathic medicine) has expanded in the West to stand almost equal to M.D. medicine while chiropractic has become a stable part of the alternatives landscape.

I am reminded of a number of occasions when I was in practice that patients came in with acute low back pain. In the military, I tried referring ailing soldiers to Physical Therapy with very little to show for their visits. On one occasion, I took a young black soldier who was experiencing persistent and severe lumbago into the nearby town of Manhattan, Kansas, and got a chiropractor to work on him gratis. Just the thought of a white officer taking an enlisted black man to a civilian chiropractor on our own time must have helped ease the young man's discomfort. Unsurprisingly, my foray into the city did not sit well with my orthodox supervisor, the Division Surgeon.

Even during my time in medical school, I had the gumption and naivete to take a patient to an osteopath. I ran into Ben and Emily Davis (see Working in Pain) at the Hermann Hospital some time after I left the Pain Service. Ben continued to have severe inguinal pain and wasn't happy with Dr. Duval's big needles. One of the Davises asked, "Do you know an acupuncturist?"

Before the day was out, I escorted them to the nearby office of Reginald Platt, D.O. Dr. Platt spent a generous amount of time with

Ben on that and several succeeding days, using every modality and approach at his disposal. The Davises stayed in a motel close at hand and visited Platt once or twice daily. Reggie gave Ben gentle osteopathic adjustments and acupuncture treatments as well as analgesics. Davis still got needles but nothing like the huge ones he had dealt with at the Pain Management Service. Sadly, the benefits of Dr. Platt's intense efforts were short-lived and modest.

Ben continued making the rounds until he found his way back to another hospital. The neurosurgeon, who previously had refused to operate on Ben, proceeded to do a neurectomy, cutting the nerves into his groin. Eventually, Davis had a cordotomy - partial transection of the spinal cord - even while brain surgery was being contemplated. But of a sudden, Mr. Davis died of "unrelated" complications. I clearly remembered Ben's words: "I'm going to beat this pain - or die trying."

By the time I was in civilian practice at the A.R.E. Clinic, I had been introduced to numbers of alternative treatments for pain and injury other than powerful drugs, anesthetics, and surgery. I had studied and apprenticed with hands-on practitioners. But, I had only begun and felt entirely inadequate when a patient came in with the likes of low back pain.

I remember an auto mechanic up the street from the Clinic who came in one day with pain in his back which had him bending over like an old man. The best I could do for him was write a script for a muscle relaxant and suggest he see a chiropractor. I apologized, "I wish I could do more."

All these experiences made me wonder about how limited I and other physicians were in similar circumstances. Practically all I was trained to do was order tests, hand out pills and make referrals.

I longed to have some therapeutic talent which might directly help to alleviate human pain and suffering. Years back, I had begun my investigation of hands-on methods, but hadn't gotten far enough along in the process to feel comfortable with my knowledge and useful with my hands.

I had started slowly just watching students at the Texas Chiropractic College examine and treat patients with nothing but their hands. Then,

I followed Dr. Platt around on free afternoons. His office was just a few blocks north of the medical center and a lot easier to navigate than a trip to Pasadena. His practice was much more "real life" stuff than the student chiropractic clinic.

Platt's father had been an early osteopathic practitioner and his son surely carried with him many of the gifts of the first Reginald Platt's old time approach. The trim, bearded, middle-aged Platt saw a wide spectrum of patients in a small aging clinic which had the feel of the old days. His father's presence was still there. The aura of hours and hours of "working in pain" hovered about the quarters. But, Platt and his older assistant seemed immune. They knew how to touch people and yet not carry "other people's pain" home with them.

I didn't really begin to understand adjustments (chiropractic) and manipulations (osteopathic) until I went away again from the Texas Medical Center for another senior elective. I managed to get the Assistant Dean of our medical school to okay a month at the Kirksville College of Osteopathic Medicine.

I had already established a correspondence with Dr. Paul Kimberly, Chairman of the Department of Osteopathic Theory and Methods. It was he who directed me to Reginald Platt and then quickly opened the door to my visit to KCOM.

I took a train to Kirksville, Missouri, arriving on New Year's Day 1977 and shared a room with a freshman student from upstate New York on the top floor of the Atlas Club. The osteopathic students were a different lot from the allopathic bunch I knew. The DO (Doctor of Osteopathy) students were more like hometown folks. That was easily explained because they were spending four years in a small town environment (about 15,000 vs. Houston about 1,500,000) and many of them would go on to become small town practitioners. The vast majority of allopathic medical schools are situated in big cities and are associated with big university hospitals.

The abilities of manipulating DOs were touted far and wide, but even within the profession there were many who scoffed at the value of OMT (Osteopathic Manipulative Therapy). While at Kirksville, I heard the gamut of student opinions. Many freely admitted taking a spot in a

DO school only because there were no vacancies at MD institutions. (In other words, they had not stacked up to the other applicants.) Osteopathic philosophy and practice meant little to them. Others were almost born into the profession and followed in the footsteps of brothers and uncles, fathers and grandfathers. They seemed to be "dyed in the wool."

My month's introduction and indoctrination consisted of attending freshman and sophomore OMT lectures and labs, participating in an upper level course in cranial osteopathy, and spending hours in the KCOM library with books, manuals, and monographs. Although I had had a whiff of chiropractic and a taste of osteopathy before my journey to Kirksville, my elective still allowed me only a nibble at a philosophy and modality which is relatively broad and inclusive.

I remember Dr. Kimberly patiently going over the intricacies of OMT spinal anatomy, mechanics, and motion from one angle, then the next. His patience in teaching impressed me as much as his long experience and obviously deep conviction in his trade. Even now, I see Kimberly's face clearly. Bespectacled, gently smiling Paul had a full head of bushy graying hair. He was quite energetic for a man in his sixties. He had given up a lucrative private practice in Florida to return to Kirksville and teach another generation of osteopaths.

He knew OMT backwards and forwards, inside and out. His body as well as his mind and heart demonstrated his unique gifts. Kimberly's hands were extraordinarily sensitive and powerful tools. I can see them now - large bony templates covered with thinning and taut, dry and aging flesh, digits cracked by time, huge thumbs flattened and spread wide beyond their expansive nails.

Those thumbs must have palpated 100,000 spines over the course of his career. Kimberly simply passed his enormous thumbs along the spine of a student, touching the joints with the slightest of pressures to sense their state of mobility. Immediately, he visualized the spatial position of the spinal column, how the vertebral elements came to their arrangement, and what adjustments were required for correction. Dr. Kimberly side-bent, rotated, and flexed his subject into an odd contortion. Then, he ever so gently, but firmly, gave a quick thrust to an articular facet. The joint had no choice but to always return to its proper alignment. Well, almost always.

Why couldn't I sense and feel those things? I could barely detect the spinal joint hidden beneath the strong, thick muscles which cover the length of the spine. Why couldn't I see which way the joint was turned? I couldn't "see" much of anything. The joints were on the inside. I was on the outside. Those joints were like a pile of children's blocks turned and twisted in various ways and then layered over several times with thick, rubbery coatings.

The spatial arrangements seemed very far beyond my ready comprehension. The dynamics of spinal motion were awesome, not unlike the intricacies of blood circulation or nerve action. Yet, the former is much more accessible than the latter. However, I had no training in the subtleties of bodily movement in medical school. The auscultation of the heartbeat was the only dynamic function which we were taxed to learn. I must admit that its vagaries were beyond the sensitivity or interest of my "tin ears." At best, I could pick up a blatant abnormality.

I genuinely wanted to learn some of Kimberly's skills. The closest I got to understanding his osteopathic abilities came during the sessions I attended under Edna Lay. Dr. Lay was a quiet fifty-ish DO who "specialized" in cranial osteopathy and had been drawn into teaching some years back. She was made in the mold of the "real osteopaths" who dated back to the founder, Andrew Taylor Still, and to the initiator of the cranial branch of osteopathy, William G. Sutherland.

The tale wast told that while a mere student at the Kirksville school in the early 1900s, Sutherland was drawn to contemplate an "exploded" skull (all cranial bones had been separated from their neighbors, yet arranged and mounted to demonstrate their anatomical relationships) which was displayed in the school library. He became fascinated by the delicate sutures which connect the twenty-two cranial bones. His considerations suggested to him that the abutting joints of the cranium allowed for regular and dynamic movements. The long-held view of anatomists that the adult skull is a rigid box with an attached hinged flap (the jawbone) proved pure nonsense to Dr. Sutherland.

As he pondered on the gill-like appearance of the cranial sutures, he came to the conclusion that the skull had to possess some sort of rhythmic breathing motion. After his graduation and entry into osteopathic practice, Sutherland devoted tremendous amounts of time and energy to detect and understand cranial physiology. He was eventually able to identify the cranial rhythmic impulse (CRI) which is comparable to the involuntary pulsations of the heart and breathing apparatus. Dr. Sutherland also discovered specific regular movements for each cranial bone, the reciprocal connection between the skull and sacrum (the crown and the base of the spine), and the "fluid waves" which coincide with the CRI and silently permeate the whole body. Of equal importance, Sutherland and his followers were able to describe common impingements and obstructions of the craniosacral system which can be correlated with various human ailments. The Cranial Group found ways to coax injured bodies to release dysfunctions of the craniosacral system.

Dr. Sutherland became a real hero to many osteopaths over the years. But, I gathered from various sources at the college that numbers of student and practicing DOs believed that W.G. had crawled too far out on a limb. Some of those people thought there was no such thing as a cranial rhythmic impulse. Others didn't really care: "It's got nothing to do with medicine. I'm going to be a physician, not a bonesetter."

Dr. Lay's students were receptive to the concepts of cranial osteopathy and not just going through the motions. (Hers was an upper level, elective course.) On the other hand, there were a lot of raised eyebrows and shaking heads in the lab sessions when students couldn't detect the movements toward which Professor Lay directed our palpation.

As for me, I was enthralled, yet pretty much lost in the midst of the exercises. I barely remembered the names of all the cranial bones and had a hell of a time picturing them working together in a synthetic, dynamic, 3-D way. Even harder was the effort to feel the extremely minute motions which were supposedly going on in the head of the lab partner stretched out on the table before me. I felt kind of numb to those impulses and movements which "had to be there." I got distracted by the pulsations in my fingertips and in my partner's head. My own breathing and imagination got in the way. Most everything seemed to prevent me getting the feel of things. "Just touch gently and feel. Use your hands, not your brain, in this work. Don't think. Feel." Dr. Lay repeated time and again.

"Yeah! Easier said than done," I thought to myself. I'd been taxing my mind-brain for years to study and learn. I'd spent 20 years relying on my cerebral cortex and she wanted me to just detach the connections and "let the fingers to the work."

I tried. I really tried. I probably tried too hard. The best I could gather in the month's worth of classroom and laboratory sessions was small portions of the larger picture: That there is another physiological rhythm beyond the cardiac and respiratory. There is a regular essential reciprocal energy flow within the human organism. Trauma and disease can disrupt the subtle, fluid bodily mechanisms, cranial rhythmic impulses, and cranial bone movements. Cranio-sacral motions can be detected and influenced via the human touch. After most of those lab sessions, I felt pretty much the way I did around auto mechanics with whom I might have said, "I once saw a transmission." As a result of Dr. Lay's efforts, I could say, "I once felt a cranial rhythmic impulse. At least, I think I did."

Fortunately, I was to have other opportunities to learn about cranial rhythms and such. Toward the end of my tour at KCOM, I was invited to dinner by Dr. Jerry Dickey. Jerry was a young professor in the OT&M Department under Paul Kimberly. Our connection came through having the same college alma mater, Texas Christian University.

I sat at the dinner table with Jerry, Dr. Lou Hasbrouck, and their wives. Hasbrouck was another old-time DO visiting from Kansas City. After the meal, Dickey set up a portable manipulation table in the middle of the living room. "Nothing like bringing your work home with you," I thought. But, the dedicated are often like that, aren't they?

Jerry and Lou gave each other cranial osteopathic treatments. Slowly, ever so patiently, they palpated rhythms, sensed minor irregularities, and nudged internal parts and movements back into the vital stream of things. They encouraged me to "put a hand in." Jerry and Lou told me what they were sensing and what I "might feel." I nodded knowingly?

Despite my lack of real comprehension of the activity, a bit of osmosis must have taken place that evening. The triangle of people intent on sharing in a social-investigative-therapeutic setting was a refreshing experience for me. I was from that moment definitely convinced that there was something to cranial osteopathy and I had to learn more about it - some day.

My time at KCOM sped by rapidly. I left the Mecca of Osteopathy for a Capital of Allopathy - The Texas Medical Center. Before I departed, I wrote a short essay for the school newsletter, Still Kickin'. I commented on the values of osteopathy, past and present, and my hopes that the essentials of the profession might someday be accepted and utilized in orthodox medicine. I boarded a train back to Houston thinking about the irony of my visit to Missouri. The most valuable and enjoyable month of my allopathic medical school career had been spent at an osteopathic college.

Touching Experiences

Even before I took my month's elective with the Kirksville osteopathic community, I was trying to get additional hands-on training. I thought I should have a whole year of osteopathic studies. Paul Kimberly was willing to help make it happen.

However, I was indentured to the United States Army for paying my way through medical school and Uncle Sam's approval was required before I could take such an unusual step. I made a special request to the Office of the Surgeon General at the Pentagon. It took only a few weeks to find out that the powers-that-be believed my regular medical school program "sufficiently qualify you to fulfill your duties as a medical officer in the United States Army."

I was a little bummed, but hardly surprised. Still, I persisted in finding ways to learn more about hands-on therapies. I started by taking a weekend massage therapy class shortly after I arrived at the

A.R.E. Clinic. I followed other angles and took week-long courses in Neuromuscular Integration (a name palatable to both MDs and DOs) through the American Holistic Medical Association. I went to annual conventions of the American Osteopathic Association and the American Academy of Osteopathy.

John Upledger, DO, appeared at an A.R.E. Clinic Symposium and I sat in on his sessions and soon took one of his extended programs. Upledger was a middle-aged, blond-haired giant of a man. He was imposing as well as engaging. Upledger had been a researcher before and after becoming a D.O. He put a great deal of technical as well as vital energy into the investigation of Cranial Osteopathy. At the time of the program, he was still working at one of the osteopathic medical schools where he had produced a number of credible papers on his subject. Later, he wrote ground-breaking books on Craniosacral Therapy, started his own teaching institute, and created a new modality for various practitioners and a whole new profession for others.

Dr. Upledger captured his lecture audience with story after story of his experiences in the laboratory, in the operating room, in the office, and even in his own personal life. John was a talented researcher as well as an expert osteopathic practitioner, hypnotist and acupuncturist. I was taken in by the wealth of his knowledge and wide abilities. I was eager to attend his workshop.

I was hardly disappointed when I saw Upledger close up in the short course he offered. He was an excellent teacher – organized, adept at his trade, bursting with anecdotes, capable of translating ideas into practical resources. He gave us a brief overview of his field and had us jump right in to the work of feeling impulses, flows, motions, and symmetries or lack thereof. The most impressive part of his "show" was the evidences he gave of his extraordinary sense of touch. I had never seen anything quite like it before and haven't since. Dr. Upledger could put a finger on the toe of a student lying upon a table and explain the precise movements which were taking place in the subject's head. On another occasion, he was asked to check a finding on a particular person. While merely looking over the shoulder of the operator, he described the intricate actions in the patient's craniosacral system.

My main teacher in the area of touch was another osteopath who came to Arizona in midwinter 1982. Peter Armitage, DO, was an Englishman. A couple years younger than I, he was gentle, soft-spoken, reserved and always quietly calculating. He reminded me of Charles, Prince of Wales, in looks as well as manner.

Peter was bright, intelligent, and talented. He had a sense of humor, still maintaining his British aura. While he was talented at touch therapy, he was not a "touchy-feely" type. Armitage had the gift of teaching, a very smooth one. He also had the interest and the patience. I learned a great deal from him as did other students along the way.

As a teacher, Peter was quite the opposite of John Upledger with whom he had done some study. Peter was introverted, deliberate, and self-effacing. While John was dramatic, blustery, and self-promoting. Peter was a slight man with small delicate hands - and the gentlest touch. He was not accomplished and renowned like Upledger, but still had the gift.

Peter sought a position at the A.R.E. Clinic which I gladly supported, but was turned down for lack of a license. Because he was trained in Europe, he was not able to get an American osteopathic license. European osteopathy and American osteopathy are two different species. Initially, I referred patients to see Peter at his home. They invariably raved about Peter's sensitivity and help. They directed friends and family to use his services.

Still, it was difficult for an unknown and unlicensed practitioner to become recognized in the community. Peter was uncomfortable promoting himself and did it only in indirect ways. I was glad to "advertise" his talents and stimulate his practice in any way I could - even before I left the Clinic. Armitage eventually asked if he might open a "real" office with my name on the door. I readily agreed, but doubted that my name and M.D. on the shingle would be of much value.

Both of us enjoyed the occasions when I joined him as he practiced his own brand of therapeutic touch on a small clientele. It was probably bewildering for patients to have four hands working on them at one time. But once they got used to it, they seemed quite pleased. Maybe they got "twice the benefit."

Dr. Armitage saw a wide range of patients, but he seemed most successful in working with people who had suffered some sort of physical trauma. Peter endeavored to release "vectored forces" which had been driven into bodies through injury of one kind or another. It was as if he, as operator, induced the rerouting of those forces which had become stuck or clogged or damped in particular areas and parts. The energies with which he dealt were quite real, but not yet subject to simple laboratory investigation.

The subtleties which are capable of being apprehended in such work are both surprising and wonderful. Craniosacral therapy not only endeavors to release trapped forces "inside the body," but also seems to permit the realignment of forces which have been projected "outside the body." That potential was demonstrated to me in the very striking case of a disabled young woman I will call Carrie Munson.

At the time I met them through another party, the Munson family had been going through a slew of turmoil, disruption and pain. First, the elder brother suffered a neck injury in a motor vehicle accident leaving him quadriplegic. He lived on his own, but his trauma and subsequent depression affected the family deeply. Second, Mr. Munson suddenly abandoned his wife and children for another woman. He moved to distant parts. Third, Carrie and her kid brother rebelled and acted out their pains and hurts. Carrie totaled her school car. Then within a week of getting a replacement, she had another near-fatal collision.

Carrie was hospitalized at a major Phoenix medical center for almost three months with various diagnoses and complications. The physicians said she had suffered a "brain stem injury" among other things. Despite numerous setbacks, Carrie was eventually stabilized and sent home in a hospital bed to be attended by her mother, aides, and visiting nurses and therapists.

When I first entered Carrie's room, I found a frail, young woman with eyes staring vacantly in one direction. She responded only to pointed questions, otherwise rarely making intentional actions or noises. Most of the time, it seemed like "no one was home."

Carrie's arms were locked over her chest and her knees were drawn upward. During my first visit, I saw her raised from the bed and then "walked" mechanically around the room as if she were a robot. Carrie was sustained by a feeding tube which had been surgically inserted into her stomach. She had yet to recover the use of muscles required for chewing and swallowing.

The situation was frightful, but not hopeless. Carrie had already survived a host of traumas and, despite her fragility, she obviously had a vital core. She also had the wondrous strength and dedication of her mother upon which to draw. Karen Munson was convinced that her daughter would get out of bed and go back to school. She told me that the doctors were hopeful as well, but could give her no definite prognosis or timelines to go by. Actually, I suspected that having given the diagnosis of "brain stem injury" to Carrie, the physicians had limited expectations. (That may well have been another version of a "we don't know" diagnosis.)

Mrs. Munson was taking all offers, utilizing a variety of nurses, therapists, and volunteers, and following up on many suggestions. When I indicated that my associate, Dr. Armitage, might be of some aid, Karen was receptive to his gratis therapeutic efforts.

Peter was interested as well and drove with me to the Munson home on an appointed day. After introductions, Dr. A. intently went to work. According to Peter's readings, Carrie's whole craniosacral system had been disrupted by the mishap. He recognized all sorts of "lesions" which demanded attention. Peter visited Carrie on a number of other occasions with me looking on. I put my hands on a couple of times, but was thoroughly confused by what I felt - or thought I felt.

I couldn't understand Carrie's situation from a strictly physical or even a craniosacral view. But, I came up with my own fairly plausible explanation based on an energetic perspective. First of all, I believed that Carrie's subtle (etheric) body had been displaced from her physical form - or maybe it was the other way around. The accident basically propelled Carrie "out of the body." She was either having a struggle getting back in or just taking her time about the whole thing - maybe both.

Secondly, Carrie's hold on the body was at the level of the heart about which her arms were tightly clasped. I sensed she was not letting go, but hanging tight. At the same time, I suspected that Carrie had some deep fear of returning to the "real" world because of all the recent trauma which had touched her and her family. It seemed to be a twisted case of adolescent existential ambivalence.

There came a breakthrough several weeks after Carrie came home and days after Peter and I stopped visiting. Whether or not Peter's efforts helped nudge her back in the direction of life, I don't know for sure. I'd like to think so, but ... After the turning point, Carrie made a then speedy and dramatic recovery. Quite amazingly, she returned to graduate with her high school class.

I have been fortunate to use touch, not just osteopathically and therapeutically, but also in simple human ways of reaching out to connect. Some time after my first contacts with John Upledger, I had an experience with a patient at the Clinic which I can best describe as delightful. I owe much of the credit for the happening to Upledger and the ideas he offered for my consideration during the Symposium.

On call one evening for the Clinic, I was asked by the answering service to contact Mrs. Johanson. My phone call was intercepted by her husband who said that she was having some breathing trouble. He thought it best that his wife be seen right away. I readily agreed to meet them at the Clinic as soon as they could make the drive.

I walked the few blocks to the Clinic and was there when Mr. and Mrs J. arrived. Lena Johanson, a stout middle-ager, was wheezing and sputtering a fair bit, but otherwise seemed her usual anxious self. I had only encountered the lady on a couple of routine visits previously, but didn't need to refer to her thick chart to feel at ease consulting with her.

Lena was a sixty year-old woman of obvious Scandinavian extraction who carried a slight accent. She also possessed a long medical history which included two operations, recurrent asthmatic attacks, high blood pressure, and obesity. Lena was short and round. Despite her afflictions, Mrs. J. was sweet, jolly, and rather childlike. She lived with her husband somewhere on the eastern edge of Phoenix toward the mountains.

While her husband waited in the lobby, I took Mrs. J.'s vital signs and tried to settle her down. She was breathing rapidly and noisily, but it was obvious that she was in no danger. I eventually moved her to an examination table, making her as comfortable as possible. As I did, I asked questions and tried to get a handle on her sudden asthmatic attack. When Mrs. J. was suitably reclined, I suggested that she rest while I placed my hand over her abdomen.

While I sat there, a number of things occurred spontaneously. Lena began to relax and her breathing eased. She sputtered and sighed and then seemed to shift into a different gear. I noticed the changes, but held on until the notion popped into my awareness that Mrs. J. was afraid of something. I asked, "I'm wondering if you might have been worrying about something recently?"

Lena quickly responded, "How did you know? My husband read something from the newspaper which really bothered me. I've been stewing about it ever since. The paper said that they have discovered cracks in the dam above where we live. Someday, the dam may break and all its water come flooding out. We might get caught in its path. Oh, my! It really scares me!"

I probed a little further and Lena added, "Lars thinks we're probably safe for ten or twenty years. but I'm worried just the same. I guess I've gotten myself all worked up over it. Lars told me not to worry. He says, 'If it happens tomorrow, we'll be okay. We have a boat.'"

Lena's apprehensions were not fully allayed because of the boat that Lars had "moored" into the backyard. Nor would her worries go away with any of my brief counsel. But, by simply touching, waiting, and listening, Lena's asthmatic spasms slowly dissipated and her state of being was considerably improved - at least for the moment. I was pleased and so was Lars. Lena didn't seem to know what to think - in more ways than the obvious.

In retrospect, I imagine that Mrs. J. was anticipating an injection or some other medical intervention when she arrived at the Clinic. I sent her home with some recommendations about using her regular medications as well as a few words of support. I told Mr. J. of my sense that Lena's anxiety was a key factor in the asthmatic attack. "Be careful what items you read out of the paper to your wife." Lars laughed.

I remember working with another patient some months later. A husky 30+ year-old man appeared in the company of his wife. He was in distress because of intermittent, severe flank pain for the past 72 hours. He had been diagnosed as having a kidney stone at a hospital emergency room and was given narcotic analgesics for home use. The relief he gained was only temporary. His pain returned quickly, but was compounded by a narcotic fog.

The young man was quite aware that he was then passing through some critical moments in his life - losing a job, relying on his wife to pay bills, wondering which way to turn in reorienting his career. It was encouraging that he could see that his "passing a kidney stone" was an outer manifestation of all the subjective changes he was going through. The patient was quite clear and expressive about his fears and worries. His wife was right there with him. The whole session - the one and only contact I had with the couple - was almost magical.

After hearing his story and considering his situation, I realized that I had little but my hands to offer him. I made some short and rather fumbling explanation about using therapeutic touch as an aid for his problem. He readily agreed to recline on the treatment table as his wife nodded her ascent. I started with some general relaxing techniques at his head and neck, and worked my way slowly toward his feet. I had no great expectations for my efforts. I merely hoped that we could ease the young man's discomfort.

I eventually moved down to his abdomen, placing one hand over his solar plexus and the other under his mid-back. I maintained that position for some time in the stillness of the room. Gradually, there came a pulsating, throbbing vibration between my hands. I could tell that the patient and even his wife were aware that something was going on. I held on while the throb turned into a momentary glow and then slowly faded away. I took a few more minutes to complete the contact.

When the patient sat up, his pain was entirely gone and there were tears of relief in his eyes. His wife was at his side. We had some good-bye hugs after sharing final words. I saw neither man nor wife again. While it appeared that my hands had been a benevolent aid to the pained patient, it may have been I who received the greater gift.

Holy Presence

The dimensions of healing, as of life, are myriad. Likewise, the dimensions and forces which can be contacted through the touch are numerous. Yet, the tendency is for an operator to fall into a rote pattern of working with patients.

No two people are identical. No two bodies, well or ailing, are the same. That makes each therapeutic meeting unique. With such an entree as hands-on therapy, there is no limit to what a practitioner (or layperson) may co-create with another person.

The body and the being are not just the crossroads of material, physical forces. That has been demonstrated in many traditions through the ages and now again through the investigations of modern physics. Theoretical physics may some day help open more doors to begin to reveal the next layers of the human onion. Eventually, we will "see" that the dimensions of life are not just physical, but are also energetic, emotional, mental, spiritual, social, environmental. Each being is an intricate, magical vortex of forces which spiral in and through us to connect us to the rest of the world.

Anyone who touches another human being or even comes close to one - contacting the other's aura - makes connections with that person and engages in a transfer/exchange of energies, however unknowingly. The touch therapist is peculiarly involved in such a process. While many ot the effects of his/her work may be inapparent or invisible, the hidden forces which meet in healing encounters are surely extraordinary. Dimensions of mind, heart, and soul can be quickened and transformations set in motion. Amazing things CAN happen when one touches or is touched.

Often baffling to me have been the occasional results of placing my hands upon or near a friend in an attempt to bring rest or relief. I have sat meditatively and watched for long times as they were transported to different times and spaces, entered altered states, or just drifted into periods of sleep. Fortunately, such occurrences were quite uniformly freeing and uplifting. Sometimes, the subjects "returned" with wide-eyed gazes, grateful sighs of release, hard-to- tell experiences.

I had my own "release" following the trauma of a sudden, but not totally surprising auto mishap. For many years, I was subject to car karma. I have had few illnesses in my life, but I have dented many other vehicles.

I have only met one person who freely admitted to having more motor vehicle accidents than I had. Russell Thomas, a Phoenix psychologist, and I once got into a conversation about our driving records. We counted them and he beat by an incident or two. He even admitted to running into another vehicle in the middle of the Kalihari Desert in Africa!

At the time of my latest event, I had been strained by a number of relationships. I was being the "nice guy" and taking care of more people than was healthy for me - or probably even them. But, I was relatively oblivious until ...

I left a lunch meeting in Phoenix and drove east toward my office. I don't recall what was on my mind at the time, but it was undoubtedly clouded by some of the strange comings and goings.

I attempted a left turn at a busy Phoenix intersection - one of those which has a left turn lane but no separate signal for the turn. When the traffic temporarily cleared in the oncoming lanes, I nonchalantly and incautiously started my left turn. I seemed to be magnetized into the intersection.

Suddenly, a car appeared racing toward me as I continued what felt like a slow-motion pace toward Camelback Road. While I thought to myself, "Oh, no! Not again!," the oncoming car smashed into the passenger side of my vehicle causing it (and me) to rotate and skid into another automobile. In the midst of all the action, I was aware that there was some overriding impulse behind the scenario. There was a surreal sense to the whole moment - until I got out of my car and surveyed the situation.

The results of the "accident" were damage to three vehicles, a traffic ticket for "failure to yield the right-of-way," a bruised ego and a disoriented state of mind. I accepted the ticket sheepishly and tended to arrangements for automobile repairs. I brooded for some days over the significance of my "failure to yield" and eventually came to some helpful conclusions on the subjective aspect of my problem. I was also fortunate to have a colleague who could tend to some of the physical effects of the mishap.

I put my body into the hands of Peter Armitage. Actually, Peter noticed - without my mention - my "disjointed" state of being a day or two after the incident. He offered to help me with his touch. "Come in here and stretch out on the table."

As I lay still upon his treatment table, his hands joined energetically with my body. He sensed the movement of forces which jarred my body and being in the "accident." Peter coaxed or cooperated with a release of the forces which I had absorbed during the accident. In a few moments, my bodily energies seemed to shift, balance, equilibrate. Soon, I was "back." Well, mostly so.

In the midst of that single session, I relived the sensation, motion, and emotion (anger at myself) of the accident. In addition, as I passed through a replay of the episode while on his treatment table, I was aware of the releasing of the energies which had been entrapping me. To my relief, I stepped down from the table with "lightened" energy and a fresh view of the mishap and the moment. My disorientation lifted like a veil and I subsequently set about "the righting of the way" in my life.

With just a modest amount of reflection, I realized that "failure to yield" was not my problem. Rather I was yielding too much of myself. I had really been letting people "run over me." The nice guy approach is not always the best. I came to the conclusion that The Big G didn't always send people into my life for the benefit of my medical talents or personal comfort. I realized that I wasn't capable of handling everyone's problems. Some of the people and patients who came to me needed to be told, "No. You need to do for yourself first. Get motivated and moving. When you do, some one will be ready to give you an extra hand along the way."

Life is complicated and so are illness and injury. Physicians and patients may want to simplify problems and make them purely physical ills. But, no such animal exists.

I learned and gained many things from Dr. Peter Armitage. One more thing he shared with me was his admiration for Rollin Becker, one of his osteopathic colleagues who worked in Dallas, Texas. I never had the opportunity to meet Dr. Becker, but have read some of his writings (thanks to Armitage.) Four brief excerpts from his article on *Diagnostic Touch* may fit in usefully here.

"There are always three problems every time a patient enters your office. There are the patient's ideas and beliefs of what he considers his problem to be; there is the physician's concept of what he considers the patient's problem to be; and, finally, there is the problem of what the anatomical-physiological wholeness of the patient's body knows the problem to be."

"Anatomical-physiological" wholeness ought to be expanded from the body to include other layers of energy, emotions, mind, soul. I believe Dr. Becker would make allowances.

"To sum it up as simply as possible, the patient is intelligently guessing as to the diagnosis, the physician is scientifically guessing as to the diagnosis, but the patient's body knows the problem and is out-picturing it in the tissues."

Two key points arise in this paragraph:

• Believe it or not, your physician is almost always GUESSING about your complaint or illness. Both patient and physician make GUESSES about illness and injury. One intelligent and the other scientific (so-called).

• The patient's problem is "outpictured" into the tissues. Again, we might want to think about the other layers of the human being. We might say that "the problem of the whole being is outpictured into the body."

"You learn to feel into the heart of the patient's problem from a still-leverage point that allows the functions and dysfunctions of the patient to be reflected back into your touch and feel. The first step in developing this depth of feel and touch is to reevaluate the patient from the third problem standpoint, just what does the patient's body want to tell you? Take the patient's story and opinion and set it aside, take your opinion and diagnosis and set it aside, then let the patient's body give you its opinion. Place your hands and fingers on the patient in the area of his complaint or complaints. Let the feel of the tissues from the inner core of their depths come through your touch and read and 'listen' to their story."

Dr. Becker and his talented osteopathic colleagues learn how to "touch and read and listen to the story" of the body. This is a huge and sometimes sufficient step to bring useful changes and relief to ailing patients. But generally, it is only an early step in gathering together the complete package required for healing. Healing is dependent on the creation or re-creation of wholeness of the being, not just the body.

"At the very core of total health there is a potency within the human body manifesting it in health. At the very core of every traumatic or disease condition within the human body is a potency manifesting its interrelationship with the body in trauma or disease. It is up to us to learn to feel this potency. It is relatively easy to feel the tensions and stresses of trauma and disease as they are manifesting this pattern of trauma of disease. But within these manifesting elements there is a potency that is 'able to control or influence; having authority or power.'"

Becker suggests that the 'potency' of disease and injury can be detected with the hands. This prompts further thoughts.

• That 'potency' can be redirected toward health and healing.
• The hands of the operator are extensions of brain, mind and heart.
• A true healing interaction between patient and practitioner surely calls out cooperation at inner levels of mind, heart and soul.

Practitioners like Rollin Becker and Peter Armitage and John Upledger suggested to me that there are true and deep possibilities for understanding and healing human ills. But, I kept coming back to the "layers of the human onion." Surely, we are not just bodies, however intricately and delicately we are perceived, scoped and examined.

Dr. Richard Selzer brought those deeper possibilities more clearly to mind in a story he wrote for Harper's Magazine (Jan. 1976). It was later collected into a book called *Mortal Lessons*. Dr. Selzer, a surgeon and partner of Bernie Siegel in Connecticut, told of how he joined some of his colleagues on a June morning at 6:00 for hospital rounds led by Yeshi Dhonden, Personal Physician to the Dalai Lama.

"At precisely six o'clock, he materializes, in a sleeveless robe of saffron and maroon. His scalp is shaven, and the only visible hair is a scanty black line above each hooded eye." Dr. Dhonden had spent the previous two hours preparing himself in praying and meditating, etc.

A patient with a long-standing chronic illness had been chosen by the staff for his examination. Followed by the white-coated entourage, Dhonden entered her room and moved to her bedside. He first gazed at the woman and then fixed his eyes above her form for a time. Selzer detected not the slightest outer clue of her disease.

"At last he takes her hand, raising it in both of his own. Now he bends over the bed in a kind of crouching stance, his head drawn down into the collar of his robe. His eyes are closed as he feels for her pulse. In a moment he has found the spot, and for the next half hour he remains thus, suspended above the patient like some golden bird with folded wings, holding the pulse of the woman beneath his fingers, cradling her hand in his. All the power of the man seems to have been drawn down into this one purpose. It is palpation of the pulse raised to the state of ritual. From the foot of the bed, where I stand, it is as though he and the patient have entered a special place of isolation, of apartness, about which a vacancy hovers, and across which no violation is possible. After a moment the woman rests back upon her pillow. From time to time, she raises her head to look at the strange figure above her, then sinks back once more. I cannot see their hands joined in a correspondence that is exclusive, intimate, his fingertips receiving the voice of her sick body through the rhythm and throb she offers at her wrist. All at once I am envious -- not of him, not Yeshi Dhonden for his gift of beauty and holiness, but of her. I want to be held like that, touched so, received. And I know that I, who have palpated a hundred thousand pulses, have not felt a single one."

The consultation was at an end except for Dhonden's examination of a specimen of the patient's urine. He whipped the liquid with two sticks for some minutes until a foam was raised, then bowed over it and inhaled the odor three times.

Dhonden turned to leave as the patient called to him as she touched her wrist with her other hand, "Thank you, doctor." Dhonden had not spoken a single word during the session.

The group repaired to a conference room where Yeshi Dhonden began to speak in soft Tibetan syllables which were translated simultaneously thereafter. "It is like the chanting of monks. He speaks of winds coursing through the body of the woman, currents that break against barriers, eddying. These vortices are in her blood, he says. The last spendings of an imperfect heart. Between the chambers of her heart, long, long before she was born, a wind had come and blown open a deep gate that must never be opened. Through it charge the full waters of her river, as the mountain stream cascades in the springtime, battering, knocking loose the land, and flooding her breath."

A professor announces the medical diagnosis: Congenital heart disease. Interventricular septal defect, with resultant heart failure. (The woman had a hole in the wall of her heart from birth.)

Dr. Selzer concludes, "Here then is the doctor listening to the sounds of the body to which the rest of us are deaf. He is more than doctor. He is priest."

Little more can I add except to say that Selzer himself a surgeon, must be one of the Wise ones. And, two such holy physicians can be multiplied into many.

House Calls

Medicine often equates with doctors and their offices, clinics and hospitals. But as noted some chapters back, drawing patients to those facilities creates clearly abnormal situations. People get sick at home, at work, on the road, in school, etc. But, medical investigation almost totally ignores "the scene of the crime."

A physician's history-taking very commonly addresses little or nothing with regard to the environment in which the patient's illness arises. So much is lost, missed or ignored simply because patients "go to the doctor" instead of the doctor going to patients, as in days of yore.

A parishioner told me the following story many years ago when I did some interim pastoring in small town churches. Thinking that ministry might make a more suitable profession for me after leaving medicine, I pointed in that direction for a time. The story brings the two - medicine and ministry - together with a number of multi-dimensional implications. It goes like this:

Over a hundred years ago, there was a kindly and fastidious, aging family doctor who lived in a small rural town. He was approaching retirement age and wanted to find a young physician to share some of the load in his latter years. Furthermore, he was concerned that his patients should have good care when he hung up his stethoscope and passed on his practice.

So, the gentleman took on a recent medical school graduate as his associate and potential partner. The young fellow was eager, but lacking in confidence as well as experience. The senior regularly and continually took moments to teach and mentor his new charge. His constant mantra was about OBSERVATION. He reiterated time and again, "Observation is the key to good medical practice."

Shortly after the new graduate arrived, two house calls were appointed on a particular day. The elder physician took the young man aside and lectured him, "Now, the house call is a wonderful thing because you, the visiting physician, have so many extra opportunities to gather information, clues, hints, etc. Your powers of observation can gather rapid and very valuable information which is much more difficult to ascertain in the office setting. Now, I want you to remember that as we go out on rounds today. The key is to Observe, Observe, Observe."

The medics gathered their equipment and took a carriage to make their house calls. As they neared the first home, the elder said, "I shall take the first call. You keep a close eye on me and the patient and, by all means, cultivate your powers of observation."

The two walked up to the house with the older man in the lead. He knocked on the door and the two were quickly led to the parlor where they found the lady of the house resting on the sofa. The lead physician introduced his new assistant and proceeded to do a brief history and a cursory examination. Within a few minutes, he brought himself up to attention in front of his patient and announced, "Madame, I perceive that you have been eating too much candy. I believe you know what I mean. You pay heed and take these tablets. You should be well in a few days."

After the physician dispensed the medication and gathered his tools into his bag, the doctors departed to their carriage. En route, the younger addressed his mentor. "I'm sorry sir, but I missed it. The diagnosis, I mean. I never heard that diagnosis in the classroom, hospital or clinic during training. Please explain."

"By all means," said the elder. "If you had been observant, you would have noticed that the good lady had a number of candy boxes - empty candy boxes - lying around her living room. That clue added to her retinue of digestive symptoms made it quite clear that she had been eating too much candy. Ninety percent of the diagnosis was made simply through observation. Do remember that when you take your turn."

The medical pair drove on to the next house. The younger medic took the lead and marched up to the door giving it a solid knock. There was no response. So, he knocked again and again. Eventually, a shaky voice called from the rear of the house, "Come in."

The gentlemen made their way into the lady's bedroom where the young M.D. introduced himself and his mentor. The patient was found propped up on some pillows, appearing a little flushed and flustered. Nonetheless, the new graduate proceeded with his history and examination which were both more involved and meticulous than the older physician's had been an hour earlier. While very methodical, the young man appeared nervous on a number of occasions, but no more so when, nearing the end of the examination, he dropped his stethoscope on the floor. He sputtered a bit as he hurriedly retrieved his precious tool.

Within a few moments, he brought himself upright and turned to his patient, saying, "Madame, I do perceive that your problem is too much religion. I quite suspect that you know what I mean. Now, I wish you to take these few tablets and mind your habits. You will certainly recover shortly."

The two colleagues quickly repaired to their carriage. As they did, the elder stopped his young assistant, saying, "Now, this one is on me. My dear boy, I have never in forty years made any such diagnosis. Your bedside manner and medical skills appeared quite satisfactory, but your diagnosis is surely perplexing. Can you help me understand how you came to that conclusion/"

"Why, yes sir, I will gladly do that. I must admit to you that I was trying to keep all your instructions and my own training in mind during the consultation. And very honestly, even with all my knowledge and an observing eye activated, I hadn't much for clues to the lady's disturbance until the very end of our encounter.

"As I was feeling stumped, my nerves got the best of me and I dropped my stethoscope on the floor. When I bent over to retrieve it, I turned my head and peeked under the bed. Well, my powers of observation did right by me. There and then, I recognized the minister of the local church lying on the floor. My diagnosis was sound and sure. The lady clearly had too much religion."

This story suggests a number of things worth considering:

- The home environment is tremendously important to health. How little do most people, including physicians, know about what goes on behind the front door of a person's home. Only friends, neighbors and rarely social workers know such. And often, they only get the "vacuumed and sanitized" version.
- Diet and nutrition, eating habits and meals or lack thereof certainly have impact on health and potential to cause dis-ease. Physicians know miniscule amounts about this general area of life. They also miss much other useful information because they don't see their patients in real life

situations.

- Religion and sex and politics, things we are all supposed not to discuss, should be part of a physician's survey. They certainly affect most every patient's life and their health as well.

Many physicians pride themselves in being "thorough." Patients often comment on that quality in their practitioners. But how can they really begin to understand the people they claim to serve until they get a more expansive sense of their patient's real life and home environs.

Wise Physicians recognize the importance of the world outside their offices and the hospital. Illness doesn't begin there and rarely ends there. The future of medicine must develop more respect for the home as well as more room for House Calls.

Family Practice

House calls are not about to soon become major parts of medical care in the modern world. They are, however, making a recovery with some physicians in some areas of the western world.

What is easily and immediately possible is the more frequent involvement of physicians in their communities, with patient families, as neighbors and friends, teachers and mentors. In the present situation, medics are often overworked and overly focused on repairing and fixing patients, and sometimes themselves. If they were to expend some of that energy and time in improving their environments, they might see surprising benefits: less illness and dis-ease, healthier people AND fewer patients.

Fewer patients might not be so good for their wallets and bank books, but would certainly be better for their surroundings and the whole world. Promotion of health, education of the population, improvement of the environment are all beneficial to everybody.

The latter should be a guiding principle for a Frugal Physician. Regardless of a patient's medical state, a prudent doctor seeks to enhance his/her overall health and welfare, teach general principles and simple home health concepts, and support a positive mental- emotional and social-spiritual community.

Just treating emergencies, plugging leaks and repairing damage done is clearly near-sighted and falls short of the mark. Health is so much bigger than doctoring, healing far beyond regular medicine. "Where there is no vision, the people perish." (Proverbs)

Starting postgraduate medical training in a Family Practice residency, I took advantage of some opportunities to relate to fellow human beings not only in the clinic and hospital but also in home settings and beyond. I fondly remember old retired sergeant Henry Baxter who was my patient off and on for much of my internship year. He followed me or I followed him around the hospital in his latter days.

While I was working with Dr. Owens (see Cut to Cure), Sergeant Baxter was admitted for care of an ulcer on the heel of his left leg. I had already encountered Baxter before on the Medical Service which gave me a leg up, so to speak.

Owens clearly "took charge" of the situation - at least for a time. He "prescribed pills" (antibiotics) and proceeded to debride the patient's wound in a rough and hurried manner. Elwood carved away tissue - some dead and some quite vital - on the edge of the wound without, to my view, the benefit of sufficient local anesthetic or proper explanation to the patient.

Mr. B. rebelled. Dr. O. became angry and defensive. Mr. B. wouldn't bow to Dr. O.'s surgical "care." I was forced, but not unhappily, in between the two, the surgeon handing over main responsibility for Mr. B.'s treatment. Owens tried to forget about "that distasteful old man." While on the "heels" of our previous contact, Mr. B. and I got along chummily.

Henry Baxter was a bit crazy at times, in part, because of medication. But, he certainly had a funny side. He was mostly bald and had a face bloated from cortisone. With all his ails, he still put on a show at times. He spoke with an almost British accent and reminded me of Winston Churchill.

Our chummy relations helped out dramatically as did "cutting" back on debridement of his wound. Instead, we hooked up a TNS (Transcutaneous Neuro Stimulator) unit to his leg to try to stir the vessels, nerves and life forces to his extremity.

In retrospect, it is hard to reckon what most helped with Mr. Baxter. Personal and friendly contact or electrical stimulation or trying something different or the passage of time or God's grace.

To put things in perspective: the vast majority of physicians and surgeons (including Dr. Owens) have specific knowledge and valuable technical skills. But, the nuances of life, the differences in human beings, the factor of time and the flow of body energies make for a host of forces with which we all must deal. Wise Physician create ways to cooperate with their patients in practical and sympathetic as well as competent.

By the time we came together, Mr. Baxter had been treated very aggressively for his diagnosis of metatstatic prostate cancer by the removal of body parts including his pituitary gland as well as his prostate. The former is a major intrusion into a person's head, glandular system and consciousness. He got leg and other ulcers and went off his nut a few times. I sat with him and listened to his stories and some of his hallucinations, visited him at home, drove him to the Post Exchange to go shopping. I eventually took his wife into my family practice panel so she could have more regularity in medical care.

I also took myself to Sergeant Baxter's funeral. His wife Paula (Leopoldine), Henry's Austrian war bride, used to send me cards and pecan cookies and Christmas every year from her Alabama home. When I left for my next duty station, she sent me off with a Red White and Blue afghan which has covered my couch for years.

Working with the Baxters and others really helped to put Family into my Family Practice Residency. Relocating to Arizona, this physician found other real, old-fashioned ways to touch at least a few people's lives. I admit I may have been a bit naive in some of my dealings with them. I tend to trust people too much, rather than not enough. Better to error on the side of goodness.

I was on duty at the A.R.E. Clinic late on a Friday afternoon when I was introduced to Jesse Chrisman. An extraordinary creature with a sad past and questionable future. Unfortunately, I lost touch with Jesse long before I left Phoenix. His row to hoe likely has not been much better than the one he was working on in the 80s.

I had the clinic pretty much to myself that afternoon. As I was getting ready to round things up for the day and the week, one of the receptionists told me that there was a young man in a treatment room waiting to be seen. "I hope it's all right. We found him passed out on the lawn. It's really hot outside and we were concerned for him." The young women coaxed him from the lawn into the building for medical attention.

Jesse didn't seem ill or injured. He was an anxious, hyperactive, and talkative 25-year-old man in a shirtless, bronzed and dirty body. Despite his hangover and ragged appearance, partly toothless smile, and frequent, "Thank you, Jesus," I was not put off by Jesse in the least.

Jesse was straightforward. He told me he only had a small pain in his side. He had just been "resting" on the lawn. "I only need a little money to get some food and a place for the night."

I was also direct. "I won't give you any money, but you're welcome to spend the night in my house and share my food."

"Thank you, Jesus."

After closing up shop, J. C. and I walked to my place. Just a couple blocks east on Fairmount. Our first task was to get him clean. I threw his clothes into the trash while he sat with the water running in the bathtub. Jesse's body needed a real scrubbing and as he wasn't the best shape to do it, I lent a vigorous hand to the job. It took two tubs of fresh water and plenty of soap and shampoo to get him even close to clean. Afterwards, the tub itself was in need of its own scrubbing. To complete the process, I dug up clothes for Jesse to put on. He then looked near to "normal." Actually, he looked good cleaned up and with a broad smile, despite the missing teeth.

Thereafter, I rustled up some plain vegetarian food which Jesse engulfed happily. "Thank you, Jesus." It took me some time to convince him that his religious rhetoric would get him no extra points with me. We passed an otherwise quiet evening, especially as I didn't own a TV or even a radio at the time. Chrisman turned in early and slept until midday. When I gathered that he was in no hurry to leave, I offered him the option of staying as long as he remained sober. Jesse again accepted.

Jesse's story was pretty simple, at least on the surface. He came from a broken home. His father had either died or absented himself from the family which lived in Grand Junction, Colorado. His mother still resided there, but the Chrisman boys had long since parted for distant places. Jesse and one of his several brothers hit the streets in their early teens. They did alcohol and drugs of all kinds - but mostly alcohol. Jesse made it to Phoenix in the late 70s and stayed because the weather was favorable for street people like himself. He worked on occasion, but often used the missions or asked obliging people to provide him with shelter and food.

J. C.'s only material possessions were the rags I had thrown in the dumpster. He had no wallet or ID card which reflected his lack of identity. Jesse had missed the opportunity of developing a stable persona. He viewed himself as a bum and he hallucinated, imagined, and/or believed that people called him a bum. On occasions when we were among strangers in the supermarket, Jesse would look over his shoulder toward another shopper down the row. He would stare for a moment then gain my attention with a whisper, saying, "Did you hear him? He just muttered, 'The guy's a bum. The bum.'"

It was almost funny. I could not help smiling sometimes and we even ended up laughing about his "acute sense of hearing." But, he was really quite serious.

By Monday, J. C. was well-sobered and fed, rested and wanting to stay on for a while. I quickly helped him get a job doing landscape and maintenance work at the Clinic. Jesse was paid "under the table," which he liked. He got a pictured ID card. So for a time he had a job, an identity, and a home. He also befriended old Marie, my beer-drinking, chain-smoking, Bible-reading neighbor. Jesse seemed to be accepted by the Clinic workers and responded by working hard for his modest wages.

Sadly, Chrisman was plagued by fears, anxieties and tantrums. The littlest thing could set him off. His paranoia reared its head at times and caused him real discomfort, but for the most part he filled his days with working and watching a used TV which he bought early on during his stay at my house. He had a nightly routine watching situation comedy reruns and stayed long enough to view the World Series.

And then all of a sudden (to me), one night he got plastered. After the fact, I heard that he had had some minor altercation with the office people at the Clinic. Regardless of its magnitude, Jesse had a reason and the cash to have a good drunk. On the following day, I told J. C. that if he sobered up and went back to work, I would give him another chance. He still had a job and a place to live if he wanted them.

But, Jesse repeated his performance of the previous night. When he showed up the second evening, I put his clothes in a bag and sent him away.

Chrisman returned from time to time. I fed him or just talked to him at the door. Once or twice, as my door was never locked, he dropped in and fried up some potatoes. He cleaned up after himself more or less - and left. He said he would never steal from me and he was true to his word.

There is a bit of sadness in me to be reminded of J. C. His talents were never (as far as I know) tapped, identity not developed, possibilities left unexplored.

He did live a life - a street life. His experiences must have produced some sort of gain for his soul. I write as though he were dead. He may very well be. His life expectancy had to be short.

Some months after his stay with me, I received a letter from a medical facility addressed to Jesse Chrisman at 4114 Fairmount Avenue. I had no forwarding address for him, so I saved the letter for a time. Eventually, I opened the envelope and found a medical bill for an emergency room visit he had made. The statement gave information on the services performed and charges made. The form noted Jesse to be 40 years old. (He seemed to have aged quickly.)

I feel good having opened my house (not the last time) to a stranger in need. But, I now wonder if I might have been a little more lenient or found some way to let him have his toots. After all, he had been sober, employed, responsible and happy - more or less for a month. That may have been a BIG step for him. It is hard to know how far to extend oneself.

Certainly, regular physicians know how to extend themselves technically and professionally. But, people are more than bodies and illnesses, subjects for operation and medication. Frugal Physicians learn how to meet patients as people and family. Surely, we are all FAMILY.

Home Remedies

Practically all medicine is practiced in clinics and hospitals. But, the vast majority of dis-ease and healing occurs elsewhere.

In recent generations, attention to illness and injury, death and dying has gotten transplanted almost totally to medical facilities. The natural order of things has been disturbed and displaced such as to often create more problems, pain and discomfort for people who become patients once they enter medical centers.

Ostensibly, the western world has become very successful through codes and standards, numbers and regimens that are supposed to fit most of the clientele. Drugs and surgery, laws and police, soldiers and wars work well from some angles in that model. But, many human beings don't.

We send all - or practically all - our young people to big schools so they get the SAME curriculum. People get sick and get pretty much the SAME treatment regardless of how their illnesses developed. Sicker folks are placed together into hospitals not unlike criminals who get thrown into jail together.

We - as individuals and a society - try to farm out our problems. Hand them to professionals to fix, professionals who often have similar problems of their own. We believe with enough research and expenditure of money, we can solve any problem.

But, a Frugal Physician recognizes that a huge proportion of our social and medical problems are not reducible to simple formulas, quick remedies, potent medications and sharp knives.

Obviously, all human beings are much more complicated than that. Very few of us are so fortunate to get simple diseases. Even those who do will eventually get ones of the opposite kind.

Doctors do well at treating and curing simple problems and non-diseases. They also help create dis-ease in numerous ways while they are convinced of and believe in their good works.

The problems of modern medicine are magnified:

- by making disease out of non-disease. To the point that birthing and dying are treated as diseases. Many of life's discomforts are simply the result of passing from one stage to the next.

While we recognize the changes of seasons outside us, we hugely misunderstand the changes within and make them seem as disease. We commonly make wholly natural occurrences into personal disorders.

- by turning away so broadly from the natural world toward technology, manufactured existence, and materialistic living. The society in general and probably most individuals have lost the sense of being part of the planet and connected to "All My Relations." Too many of us don't know where hamburger comes from. Other than from the supermarket.

Even farmers and ranchers are becoming shielded from nature by way of enclosed and air-conditioned tractors and trucks and combines. Crops are fertilized (with chemicals) and hybridized (in labs), sprayed with herbicides and pesticides (another form of antibiotics). The land is sapped and exploited - like many farm hands - rather than be considered at least a partner. Animals are bred and raised, inoculated and bulked up to suit the husbands' cycles not the critters.

- by assuming functions that rightfully belong to our families and our communities. Physicians and medicine - with supposed altruistic intent - have taken charge of a host of responsibilities as well as opportunities that really need to be shared with the wider society.

Disease and healing have been gradually separated off from the community. Social workers take charge of the elderly who are put frequently to pasture in sprawling nursing homes (home is often a misnomer). Child care workers intervene in family problems which may be simple effects of growth and change. Hospitals separate patients from their kin, requiring them to visit by appointments, and interfering with their involvement during very crucial moments in the lives of their loved ones.

- by ignoring the importance of the inner, spiritual life. All hospitals have chapels and chaplains, but spirituality for many is a lot broader than those two. While most hospitals were begun by religious institutions, they are now being pushed "out of the business" by profit-making corporations. Much real care and compassion and sensitivity goes with them.

The Great Physician enjoined his early followers to "preach, teach, and heal." Thus, healing was a key element of Christian churches for many centuries. But, it has been turned over to medics pretty much lock, stock and barrel. Those ministers and "church doctors" who now dare intrude onto medical turf better have malpractice insurance just like the Regular Docs.

All of these items suggest social change. Some for the good, some for the bad, and even more questionable. Most people would probably agree that the scales have been tipped out of balance, and need attention.

The western system has turned away from simple, down home, neighborly ways of relating in general and quite in particular in medical matters. This has done harm to us all.

Third world countries still use curanderos, shamans, medicine men, and other indigenous healers - definitely not university trained and board certified. Psychics, faith healers, and herbalists persist on the fringes in first world countries. But barely.

What may be even more troublesome is the loss of talents and experiences with remedies inside the family circle. The medical profession can take only partial blame for this state of affairs. Families have spread far and wide. Mothers and grandmothers often do not live in the same town or city. The ones who remain close by have been handed down little useful information to share with families and friends.

Few of the present generations know anything about the benefits of chicken soup, onion poultices, mutton tallow rubs, salt packs, oil massages, blanket wraps, etc. The rare home remedies that doctors recommend are limited usually to hydration (lots of water), cranberry juice (for "urinary infections"), vaporizers for croup. Pills and capsules, tablets and potions, nebulizers and patches are pretty much supposed to handle home needs for all people in the present age. Family involvement with these or any methods in most medical problems has become very small and little valued.

Still, we can take heed from less developed nations and cultures. We can recognize through their experiences that we are not alone, separate from each other, islands unto ourselves. Illness and injury of one affects us all. And the care of family and friends can make huge differences to the ill and injured. The closer proximity to the individual, the greater potential effect. Care is much better shared regularly and preventively, but any time can be beneficial.

As we have entered the Interactive Age via television and the internet, it might take little impetus to encourage families and friends to actively re-enter the world of healing. The treasure trove of the internet may be a useful rallying point and reference center.

The author had the good fortune to be exposed to a variety of home remedies through his studies of alternative therapies and traditions. Contact with a wide spectrum of hands-on workers also helped broaden his experience and view. Two episodes during his family practice training may help bring home the benefits of family participation, the personal touch and home remedies.

I attended both Bill and Edith Feeback in my internship. Bill was another retired Army sergeant in his late fifties. He had been a cook or mess steward. His stout, obese build made me imagine that he could have fit the part quite well. Feeback was blustery, talkative, and anxious. He was in and out of the hospital many times with angina and heart attack, stroke, and hyperventilation episodes.

His manner offended or at least irritated most everyone. I seemed to be an exception. I listened. I tried to respond to his worries and queries. Most of the time his requests were beyond my abilities to fill. And, too often they were quite unrealistic. He wanted the hospital, nurses, and doctors to do things for him and his wife which were rightly his own responsibility. Still, I listened.

Bill was rather an albatross and no one wanted Feeback tied to him or his ward. Staffers were always more than glad to see him discharged from the ward or the emergency room. Yet, if Bill wasn't a patient, his wife was and the hospital workers seemed to have even more trouble with his demands as a family member than as a patient.

Edith was diagnosed with an inoperable tumor in her chest which had spread to her brain. Her cancer was only recognized after she was admitted for work-up of her suddenly appearing seizures. By the time I met Edith, she had received maximum chemotherapy and radiation to both her chest and head. She had been sent home some days previously with a personal attendant to help Bill care for her. Her cancer doctor had shuffled her out of the hospital in part because the staff couldn't deal comfortably with her husband.

Edith showed up at the Emergency Room one evening when I was on duty. She was brought in by ambulance and I found her lying in a near-comatose state on an ER gurney. I did the usual "cursory" exam and got some basic information from Bill despite his tense and agitated state. I then made a phone call to her Attending Physician. Dr. Hermann made it quite clear to me that he had "done everything possible for this woman. There is nothing more that can be done for her. She was sent home to die."

Edith and Bill hadn't cooperated with that expectation. And, we couldn't very well send her home as she was. Hermann moaned and groaned about how overloaded he was, but said, "Go ahead and admit her for me, please." With his unspoken, yet obvious hint, I volunteered to take over Mrs. Feeback's care. Hermann was undoubtedly relieved and was quite cooperative when I consulted him later on about her case. Even while I was on the phone with Dr. Hermann, an idea was brewing in my mind to try some unorthodox methods in Edith's care.

The potential for using alternatives was now opened for several reasons. By the time I encountered Mrs. Feeback, my internship was well nigh over - I was almost home free. I was in relatively good standing in the training program after some early conflicts which put me on the short end of the stick for a time. I had even been "invited" to complete the final two years of the Family Practice Residency. I declined.

There was little to lose in trying "something different" with Mrs. Feeback. Besides, I had recently been given permission to do a clinical study on the use of castor oil packs in the treatment of minimal brain dysfunction. (See story below.) Dr. Hermann had given up on Mrs. Feeback in more ways than one and had handed over her care to me - with blessings.

I admitted her and wrote initial orders to approximate the regime she was given on her previous hospitalization. The next day I called Hermann again and asked for his okay in treating Edith with vitamins as per the work of Nobel Laureate Linus Pauling and British cancer surgeon Ewan Cameron. I intended to place her on megadoses of ascorbic acid (Vitamin C) as part of her therapy. Hermann readily agreed and even suggested adding a good dose of Vitamin E to her new plan. With his go-ahead, I ordered C and E plus multivitamins and folic acid as soon as she could swallow "pills." I added castor oil packs and mild natural laxatives to her treatment. At the same time, I gradually reduced her "drugs" - cortisone and anticonvulsants.

I involved Bill in her care by getting him to go to the commissary each day for fresh fruits - papayas, pineapples, melons which became the mainstay of her diet. (The Feebacks had been stationed for some years in Hawaii and the fruit diet suited them.) He fed and tended her carefully and comfortingly. It was great therapy for her and maybe even better for him, while it lasted. Bill was helpful and generally cooperative. He was still demanding, but reasonably pacified because his wife was being cared for and he was doing his part. However, there were bumps on the road of her treatment. And Bill felt them. He reacted and ended up in the ER a number of times because of angina and hyperventilation attacks.

Our "experiment" was successful not only from a human standpoint but also from a medical one. Edith perked up, sat up, and even started physical and occupational therapy. Her color and appetite returned. Her blood counts revived and her seizures diminished. Her bowels even worked. But, alas! Her tumor became active again. A lump appeared at the angle of her jaw and the once "frozen" mass in her chest started to grow again.

Fortunately or unfortunately, my internal medicine rotation ended and I left the program. Edith Feeback's care was assumed by a new intern. Immediate changes were made. Mrs. F.'s diet went from light fare - mainly fruits and vegetables - to standard hospital menu. Her once supposedly maximum therapy was topped off with more radiation and more anticancer drugs. The tumors again responded, but the patient lapsed into a weakened and depressed state. Edith's seizures became more frequent again. And Bill resumed his very anxious and difficult postures.

Mrs. Feeback lingered for some weeks with her latter days spent on IVs and no food intake at all. One of the residents let me know, as I was moving to my next duty station, that she lived that long because of the regime we had undertaken in the spring. I don't know what happened to Bill after his wife died. Her passing must have been extremely hard on him. He was then faced with the supreme task of caring for himself and living alone.

In retrospect, I'm not sure what I would have done if I had continued as Mrs. F.'s physician when her tumor reasserted itself. At this point, all I can think is that it must always be better to treat people than diseases. If I had it to do over again, I would have spent more time with Edith and Bill, broached sensitive topics of family and life, and even joined the fruit fest.

Castor oil packs have to be my favorite remedy - for home or hospital or anywhere. They are simple, natural, inexpensive, and comforting. They can be a bit messy, but that is part of what gives them their home remedy flavor.

They remind me of how old time druggists and apothecaries as well as modern herbalists concoct their media. Modern medicine only puts pure chemicals, necessary adjuvants and fillers into their drugs. Pharmacists and physicians forget that Nature has had its own Pharmacopoeia for eons.

Primitive peoples and indigenous healers as well as instinct-driven animals know how to find and use nature's remedies. Those items are never 99 percent pure, but combined in the substance of whole plants or organisms. They are not made in colorless, robotic, sterile factories, but in magical, life-giving realms.

Castor oil packs, simple but greasy, require only an ample supply of oil, cloth, and hot water bottle or heating pad. (The oil is relatively pure, but gets "dirtied" in the pack every time it is used and re-used. There is a story of a man who was either so in need or so taken with the packs, that he soaked the whole of his bed linen in castor oil and slept in an oily cocoon for months.)

The oil should be generously applied to two or three thicknesses of flannel large enough in size to cover the patient's abdomen from the pubic area to the rib cage. I like to slather the person's belly with a layer of the oil to begin, then put on the pack. Follow with a film of plastic sheeting and then a towel to somewhat contain the greasy effects. Lastly, some source of local heat adds to the comforting belly wrap and helps the body absorb the castor oil.

Castor oil packs, first suggested as far as I know by Edgar Cayce, are recommended for a wide variety of abdominal and pelvic complaints, and a number of systemic ones such as epilepsy and migraines. Theoretically, the castor oil is absorbed through the skin, picked up by the lymphatic system which connects with the intestinal lymphatics, and cleanses and unclogs that network. The packs are also thought to have effects upon the energy body particularly through the solar plexus. And that ain't all!

I have used COPs in the hospital and clinic environment, and recommended them for use hither thither and yon. The first time I used them in the hospital during my family practice residency, I got in deep trouble with the authorities because they weren't standard fare. After passing through a stage of probation for my blatant unorthodoxy and lying low long enough, I was not bothered when I ordered their use for

Mrs. Feeback months later.

I had my very own personal experience with the packs close to the time I worked with Mrs. F. For some days as I was turning different shades of yellow with hepatitis, I found my sleep disturbed and rest hard to come by. It took my wife to order - or suggest - castor oil packs. I slept like a baby thereafter. Within a few days during my convalescent leave, I was out planting a garden behind our apartment building.

I had one other experience with castor oil packs under "experimental" conditions in the latter weeks of my time in family practice training. A research paper was required of every resident for each year of the program. I produced my own non-standard study of Minimal Brain Dysfunction (ADD) using castor oil packs and dietary suggestions as key components following on the work of Dr. Ernest Pecci and Dr. Ben Feingold.

Interestingly, just the ADD diagnosis gives big clues to how little medics know about the "syndrome." Around forty (20 by Organic Terminology and 21 by Symptomatic Terminology) different diagnoses were used for this condition at the time. The number has undoubtedly grown over the past 30 years.

The study was of brief duration and incomplete because of my leaving the residency after the first year. But, the "preliminary findings" showed that the eight "subject children were found to have increased attention span, fewer temper tantrums, decreased activity level, improved speech patterns and school grades, and decreased number of abdominal complaints - in some children."

I didn't get to "present" my paper with the rest of the group because I was convalescing at my garden. I did turn it in, but never heard a peep from the family practice leaders. There was one thing I didn't put in my paper which was clearly important to the beneficial results which were noticed early on in the study.

That was the positive input by parents which came about with them taking the time and energy to assemble and apply castor oil packs to their children three times a week. They didn't just drop a pill into their hands, they had to attend to the children, spend some quality time with them and even touch them. How novel and nice!

After internship when I moved into work as a general medical officer, I applied castor oil packs to young soldiers with abdominal upsets on clinic premises. We didn't have flannel cloth available, but gauze pads seemed to work equally well. Since that time, I have recommended them to hundreds of people while in practice and now as an erstwhile physician.

To be honest, I'm not totally sure about the physiology of castor oil packs. But, they certainly ease symptoms without the least side effect, seem to have salutary benefit for the whole body, give patients a warm, comforting feeling, and bring people together at least for a few moments in the interests of health improvements.

Every Frugal Physician should know about castor oil packs (and other home remedies), try them on themselves, and consider adding the packs to their treatment repertory.

The Whole Works

The reader might imagine by now that we have covered most of the medical landscape. But, we are really just beginning in many ways. The Rest of the Story, as Paul Harvey might say, remains to be told.

It is time to take on "new" concepts and wider approaches as we begin to move from plain old Medicine to expansive Health and Healing. Those two simple words are really huge, though nebulous to some, and foreign to others. Scientists and physicians have spent so much time and energy, resources and research on Disease and Diagnosis. We must focus more attention on Health and Healing.

Human beings, and all living creatures for that matter, are not just collections of tissues and organs, atoms and molecules. They are wholes which are always more than the simple sum of their parts. That is obvious even to Regular Physicians. Yet, they plow ahead based on their training and their own "lights" however limited in scope they may be.

The future of medicine and the broader field of healing must find a new central emphasis. Namely HEALTH. Let's consider this Big Idea by listing some considered definitions.

- The absence of disease. This definition is a common one heard in medical circles. Many physicians believe that their job is simply to make patients comfortable and relieve them of their symptoms.

No Symptoms = No Disease = Health. But, such is very often not the case. How many people have you heard about who have gotten a clean bill of health from their physicians and had a heart attack or suddenly died while mowing the lawn the next day?

How can a physician know that a patient is disease free? Signs (test results) and symptoms hardly tell the whole story. They just give a superficial picture of things. Scans, as we shall see, only go one layer deep.

- Optimal physiology. If physicians consider health the absence of disease, medical scientists point to "normal" body functions as monitored by a slew of tests, to suggest that state. This idea points to running, aerobic training, etc. as means to build health.

But, it should be clear to most thinking folks that body building, weight training, distance running may only expand the limits of body endurance, speed, performance. Again, how many famous athletes have dropped in their tracks in their prime, bloated into balloons thereafter, or become couch potatoes in later years?

On the other hand, many people live quite healthfully with missing appendages, imperfect eyesight, bodily distortions, etc. Some humans have accomplished more in disabled bodies than many do in seemingly perfect forms.

These first two definitions are based on body parts. The reader should have a growing sense that s/he is more than body and parts. Health goes far beyond physical indicators.

- Bodily integrity. Just by looking at physical signs alone we learn that even in illness, humans generally express relative health in so many ways. Much more than we might imagine. When we feel bad, we may think that, "My whole body is falling apart." Far from it.

If we break a leg or have a stroke or deal regularly with diabetes symptoms, most of our being is still for all intents and purposes "healthy." A seeming paradox. We are still more than 99.9999 percent healthy. Most everything is working quite well, but we focus on our ills instead of our "wells." This point really needs to be brought home: to recognize the health within our frames, rather than fretting about the often small woes which we let beset our thoughts, stir our worries and point us to the doctor's office.

From the outer angle even in the worst of disease and disability, the human organism supports trillions of body cells. That's trillions; thousands of times more than there are humans on the face of the planet. Ill or well, our hearts beat billions of times during the average life. Our brains alone contain billions of active neurons. Our skins are renewed every week, stomach linings five days. The numbers and complexities of the ongoing operations within the human body and brain are truly mind boggling.

Just think about all those cells and neurons, tissues and organs, systems and networks that continue merrily along even when we are coughing, aching, or stressing out. How does the rest of our structure maintain its integrity and keep recreating itself in the midst of illness and injury?

Let's consider one more amazing health fact. Fully 98 percent of atoms in the human body are replaced within a year's time. Years ago, we used to read that the body renews itself every seven years. Scientific investigators now tell us that cycle of renewal may be less than five years. Absolutely no ailment need then last longer than one cycle of life.

Furthermore, the body is capable of changing quite rapidly and does so often without our realizing it. Which might lead us to wonder, "How long does it take a person to change his/her mind?"

- A sense of well-being. True health should include this factor. But, it is really only one part of the equation.

The problem with this definition is that human beings can delude themselves. Some tend toward manufacturing or at least magnifying illness. Others go on obliviously and pay no attention to their bodies, thinking they are invincible, made of steel, and will last forever. Different strokes for different folks. Different lessons, too.

• Living harmoniously in one's environment. This definition helps broaden health beyond the individual putting the human being in a social setting. "No man is an island," to be sure. But, to be able to function socially is only one part of the bigger picture.

And it may be of value to ponder the acid thought of Jiddu Krishnamurti who said, "It's no measure of health to be well adjusted to a profoundly sick society."

• A state of wholeness. This idea seems to stretch the definition of health to a positive and expansible limit. It allows for looking at humans as bodies with mental, emotional, social, and other attributes. And, even greater possibilities like fulfilling one's destiny, making a difference in the world, and manifesting love and spiritual gifts.

One of the author's favorite slogans is "The Whole Works." Part of getting the whole to work comes with simply recognizing that possibility. This suggests the power of the great dictum of ancient oracles, "Man Know Thy Self."

Some of the premises which support The Whole Works are:

1) The human body and being are much more than physical.
2) Human matter is human energy solidified.
3) Mind and body are intricately meshed together.
4) Spirit itself binds mind and body.
5) Dis-ease is not accidental. It is a picture of imbalance which inevitably leads back to balance.
6) Humans are generally predisposed to health and susceptible to eventual recovery and healing when sick and injured.
7) Healing is certain because humans are innately whole beings.

The Body Electric

In the coming years, the medical profession will be forced - for the betterment of all concerned - to recognize in a practical manner ideas and principles long known outside the guild and also long ignored within it. The scientific community, particularly physicists, have shown over a century ago that the material world is really energy in constant motion. That being the case, human beings must be energy in motion as well. Large portions of the general public know this simple truth which has yet to penetrate medical thinking and practice.

The present state of affairs in medicine is much like the state of things regarding our own planet until recent centuries. Most everyone including educated people in the past believed that terra firma was flat as a pancake. "Be careful not to sail to far to the West else you fall off the edge."

Yet, ancient philosophers - from Indian pandits to Chaldean, Egyptian, and Greek sages - were quite aware through study of the motion of the stars that the Earth rotates on its axis and circles the sun thus demonstrating its shape. But, it took Christopher Columbus and other explorers to "prove" the Earth to be round: a simple truth which was obvious to early thinkers.

Regarding the composition of things, the ancients knew full well that atoms were really quanta of energy. But, it took until the turn of the 20th century for physicists to "prove" that matter and energy are interconvertible. Furthermore, they demonstrated that what we perceive as solid matter is hardly such. Even the hardest of rocks - at ultra-microscopic levels - have vast amounts of space between their ever-moving electrons and nuclei.

Solid matter appears so for at least two reasons. First, solidity is a mirage like the swarm of birds we watch at a distance. So much mass moving so quickly and compactly seems to us like a solid entity. Second, our eyes have been trained to see solid matter and not energy in motion.

With that introduction, let's consider some simple concepts about the human being and energy:

- Human beings, like all other things, are energy beings. Solid as we appear, our bodies are mirages. But like Madonna, we have grown up into a "material world." We recognize aggregates and not spaces within forms, solidity not motion.

The solid material world we are used to is quite real. Others lie waiting to be revealed to us. We may one day be able to sense atoms in motion, the traces they leave and the vast spaces between them. Those spaces also contain other living forces most of us have yet to even imagine. Even now, some seers can apprehend energy and ethereal forces.

That capability may eventually be as common as technicolor vision is today. There are fascinating suggestions that we humans are even now slowly expanding our visual spectrum. Color psychologists have noted that the ancient Greeks did not have a word for blue, giving the hint that humans may have evolved the capacity to extend our spectrum of vision in the past few millennia. Further expansions of human perception are sure to occur.

This reminds the writer of the trick that optometrists use with contact lens wearers. So that patients don't have to wear lenses and reading glasses at the same time, eye doctors fit them with one lens for distant vision and the other for close-up. After a short time, the wearer's mind-brain blends the two images to see both near and far comfortably.

Today, almost the whole human race sees from one angle only. Just materially. Some day, we will have developed other "lenses" to allow vision of the physical and energetic world at the same time.

There are many medical implications from this perspective. We have seen that 98 percent of the atoms in a human body are new every year. The energetic makeup of the human form is in continual flux whether we notice or not. The constant turnover of atoms allows for rapid healing. Or change, at least.

If the change is not for the better, what is to blame? Everyone should be - theoretically - totally changeable, transformed in the course of a few years.

Part of the reason we don't heal and our bodies don't change for the better is because ill health often develops over long periods. And we often get used to our patterns of illness. Like an uncomfortable marriage, it is often easier to stay with what we know than imagine and create something new.

We are practiced at seeing, looking, being a certain way. But, maybe that need not be always so. *Miracles happen around and within us every day* (subject for another book), but we miss so many of them because we are focused on problems not possibilities, limits not potentials, disease not health, lack not plenty, fear not love.

While we seem to have limits, humans have hardly tested them. This is so, in part, because we still see the world as flat, things as solid and unchanging, life as cold and dreary, the future dark and foreboding. When will we develop the faith (knowledge) as of a mustard seed? When will we move mountains as the ancients and do greater things?

Physicians are just as guilty as the rest of us in limited, pessimistic thinking. Medics are clearly materialistic. They want solid answers and hard proof. "We don't do miracles." Doctors, despite their high calling, limit themselves and their patients by their persistent hard material view of things. They see physical bodies only. And have few clues that humans are much more. "The West studies the stomach. The East studies the soul." (*Anonymous*)

Medics try to change things materially and mechanically using chemicals and operations, the crudest of remedies. They certainly have effects but largely at the outer, superficial physical level. Quick but shallow change results, but with frequent side effects and long term ill effects. Real healing and real change must come from deeper levels. The first step in that direction will arise with the persistent, detailed study of subtle energies.

- A subtle energy body underlies the dense material body. When we can see, sense, and examine the former like we now do the latter, we will have taken the next step of real discovery for medical science. This step will begin to bring REAL SCIENCE into play in the profession.

Science really means KNOWLEDGE, not guesswork.

The outer visible, tangible human body is itself an energy body. But, it is so dense that it appears unmoving, unchanging. The outer body effectively hides the subtle body which lies within and interpenetrates it.

This energetic nature of the human form, like that of the atom, has been studied and taught in the East for many ages. Only portions of that teaching are known and used in modern times. And, those only in limited fashion.

The ancients of the West long ago wrote and spoke about the subtle body, the body spiritus, the etheric vehicle. "If there is a natural body, there is also a spiritual body." (Saint Paul) This knowledge was carried from The East which brought forth understanding of the impulses of chi and the pranic body. Practitioners of Indian Ayurveda, Chinese/Tibetan medicine and acupuncture even now use portions of this knowledge in attempts at caring for human ills.

A few of these ideas have filtered down into the present only to be kept at bay on the distant fringes of medicine. But, some of the greatest medical thinkers have clearly spoken of these aspects of human anatomy and physiology. Paracelsus and Mesmer were quite aware of them. In recent times, Walter Kilner, an early radiologist, studied the "human atmosphere." Psychiatrist Wilhelm Reich worked with "orgone energy." Harold Saxton Burr did fundamental scientific research to show that even cells have energy bodies. George Crile of the Cleveland Clinic studied the Radio-Electric Phenomena of Life. Orthopedist Robert Becker recently dusted the surface of these ideas with his book called *The Body Electric: Electromagnetism and the Foundations of Life*.

But, most of this research has been set aside and largely ignored for a variety of reasons. The simplest is that working with and understanding the energetic nature of things requires subtler levels of thinking - imagination, finesse, and intuition. A level that goes far beyond the hard technical view with which medical and scientific types can readily work.

- Study of the energy body will open doors which have long been closed to scientists and physicians intent on understanding health and disease. When only a modest investment is made in the investigation the energetic nature of living beings, huge rewards will be forthcoming.

There are obstacles in the way, just as the oil business lobbies against electric vehicles and coal companies protect against green energy. Pharmaceutical interests won't invest in studies which will elucidate the inner nature of the human frame and inevitably reveal the ill effects of their own products on the subtle bodies. And, subtle energy is not conducive to bottling.

Subtle energies will surely be found to be much like perfume. Real perfume is a volatile radiation of living creatures. People have wanted to capture the mountain air and pine forests so as to bottle them for use in the city. Approximations have been attempted. Accomplishments are still awaited.

There are ways to influence the movement and flow of body energies. But, there is unlikely to be a pill or potion, blade or operation to do it. Hard things call for hard heads and hands. Subtle calls to subtle.

The simplest way to look at the energy body is to imagine it as the body double, a template on which the outer physical is laid at birth, transformed over time, and rebuilt during periods of healing. Every vessel and nerve is underlaid by lines of force. Every organ is sustained by networks and skeins of electric light.

The energy body is thus a body of light which may be likened to a radiant cocoon for the dense physical. Until substantive human energy research in this direction takes shape, we will have to draw on hints from here and there. Stories and anecdotes and maybe even reverie will be required to ease ourselves into subtle realms.

I can't help but be reminded of Ben Davis (see Working in Pain, Good Hands). It seems clear that his problem was one that medics never would have explained and managed materially. But, they may have gained understanding by looking at it energetically.

Ben's pain was not physical. No pain is purely physical. Pain and sensation are mediated through the energy body.

Medics tried to block his pain with anesthetics with limited effect. Eventually, they severed his nerves and the spinal cord while imagining the necessity of cutting on his brain. He still had pain. How could that be? Everyone, especially neurosurgeons, knows that nerves are the channels by which pain is received and perceived in the brain!

But, that is not even half the story for Ben and the rest of us. The outer dense body is the garment, the cover, the coating. The real work goes on at subtle levels.

Thinking about the body from the energetic angle affords a whole new view and opens a wider dimension. Regular simplistic approaches of medicine to the human body continue not to work in many ills, especially regarding pain syndromes. We can think optimistically that more physicians will step up to use an energetic approach particularly in these problems. Better yet, the whole profession will begin to look at all patients and their problems from such a perspective.

This will put a different spin on a host of undiagnosable problems. Those "We Don't Know" kinds will slowly become more understandable. Medics and scientists will also be better able to fathom some of amazing physiological feats which the body accomplishes, but are often naively explained with simplistic physical and chemical concepts.

- The human heart, wonderful pump that it is, forces blood down to the feet into tiny capillaries. Every smidgen is carried back up rhythmically, practically forever. But, underlying lines of force in the energy body are the real reason such an amazing feat is possible. Blood pressures do not explain this ability adequately.
- Energy production throughout the body is supposed to be simply dependent on molecular conversions of ATP (adenosine triphosphate). Such abilities in no way can explain the extreme exercises which humans can undergo. There is not enough ATP in any body to make muscles do all the amazing and prolonged feats they can do. Even simple body activities are not knowledgeably explained under present physiological tenets.
- The human brain and nervous systems are thought to integrate the whole organism. But, the speed and agility with which humans can perform complicated "global" tasks require the much subtler and profound integration of the energy body.

- Pain syndromes, such as phantom limb pain, are said to be mediated through the sensory nerves. But, the true avenue lies in the energy body and even deeper. Phantom limb pain is explainable with understanding of the energy body, parts of which are not severed immediately when a limb is amputated from the physical form. Continuing pain and phenomena can follow the severing of a limb, regardless of medical attention. Subtle energies are implicated.
- Faith healing, hypnotism and animal magnetism can be explained through consideration of the subtle body. The dense physical may not respond where the energetic can be reached through presently unacceptable and unexplainable means.
- Recovery from brain traumas can be understood energetically. Arizona Congresswoman Giffords was shot (2011) at close range exploding her skull and destroying vast amounts of brain tissue. Physicians have no idea how her brain is now healing and rebuilding connections to allow her to recover mental function. But, the energy body simply retains the template on which her brain was first formed and is able to reconstruct it under proper conditions.

The Mind Body

Dramatic changes will occur in medicine when the energetic nature of the human body becomes part of physician thought. An even more revolutionary shift will eventuate when medics recognize what Eastern adepts have known for millennia, "The mind is not in the body, but the body is in the mind." This concept is much like the one medieval mystic Meister Eckhart championed: "The body is in the soul, rather than the soul in the body." This idea is quite simple, but the implications are profound.

Medicine has long treated human beings schizophrenically by separating bodily (somatic) problems from mental ones. Limiting the mind, placing it in a box at the top of the shoulders, imprisoning it in the brain. But, the fact is that the mind is only temporarily limited by medical thinking, works through more organs than the brain, and actually manifests through the whole body.

A field of mind, not unlike the energy body, but broader and subtler, surrounds and interpenetrates the human being. The brain is its chief but not only means of exchange with the physical form.

The general Western conception is quite opposed to the long- held Eastern view. We erringly continue to believe that the mind is strictly an attribute or function of the brain (mind = brain) and is, therefore, contained solely within the bounds of the cranial vault. Yet, there is much evidence that the mind, although limited by our use and conceptions of it, is much greater and more encompassing than we are generally aware. (How often have you heard that we use only one tenth of our mind? Maybe that is partly because we have restricted its function to the organ which sits between the ears.)

Let's consider current scientific information which indicates the mind being a greater entity than the brain:

- Lyall Watson in *Lifetide* wrote, "Each brain cell receives an average of ten thousand connections from other brain cells, and has its own molecular structure renewed completely at least another ten thousand times during its active life. The brain loses more than a thousand cells each working day, wiping out more than a trillion cross linkages in every twenty-four hours. Yet consciousness, memory and behavior continue."

- In his book *Space, Time and Medicine*, Larry Dossey discussed the research of a British neurologist, John Lorber, whose work questioned the premise that "an intact cerebral cortex is even required for normal mentation." Dr. Lorber utilized computerized brain Xrays to study hundreds of patients with hydrocephalus, a condition in which fluid gradually replaces brain tissue. "He discovered that many of his patients had normal or above-normal intellectual function even though most of the skull was filled with fluid. Normally, humans have a cerebral cortex measuring four and one-half centimeters in thickness, containing 15 to 20 billion neurons. In one patient, however, a college mathematics student who was referred to him because his physician suspected that his head was slightly enlarged, the brain scan revealed a cerebral cortex of only one MILLIMETER in thickness. Functioning, with only a tiny rim of cortical brain tissue of 1/45 normal thickness, this student proved to be gifted on standard IQ testing (he had an IQ of 126) and was normal not only intellectually but socially."

Dr. Dossey also cited exceptional cases of individuals who have had entire hemispheres removed from their cerebral cortex as treatment for intractable epileptic seizures. These procedures are commonly followed by permanent paralysis, speech disturbances, and memory or reasoning deficits. Yet, there are numbers of patients who do not react in typical ways. They recover fully and sometimes become truly gifted people.

- Surprising data has arisen from studies of the brains of famous and talented individuals. Scientists have theorized that Great Minds must have larger than normal brain size. This idea has been shown to be lacking. Consider the case of Anatole France (1844-1924), the great French novelist and Nobel prize winner (1921). He is said to have been a man of true genius and vast mental powers. Yet, autopsy showed France's body to possess a very small brain. The average cranial capacity is fourteen hundred cubic centimeters. But the skull of Anatole France, had a capacity of a mere thousand.

- Noted neurosurgeon, Wilder Penfield wrote in *The Mystery of the Mind*, "As Aristotle expressed it, the mind is 'attached to the body." The mind vanishes when the highest brain-mechanisms cease to function due to injury or due to epileptic interference or anesthetic drug. More than that, the mind vanishes during deep sleep. On this basis, one must assume that although the mind is silent when it no longer has its special connection to the brain, it exists in the silent intervals and takes over control when the higher brain-mechanism does go into action."

Penfield went on to say, "Because it seems to me certain that it will always be quite impossible to explain the mind on the basis of neuronal action within the brain, and because it seems to me that the mind develops and matures independently throughout an individual's life as though it were a continuing element, and because a computer (which the brain is) must be programmed and operated by an agency capable of independent understanding, I am forced to choose the proposition that our being is to be explained on the basis of two fundamental elements. This, to my mind, offers the greatest likelihood of leading us to the final understanding toward which so many stalwart scientists strive."

- Nobel Prize winning surgeon and researcher, Alexis Carrel, concluded in his *Man the Unknown* that, "Personality is rightly believed to extend outside the physical continuum. Its limits seem to be situated beyond the surface of the skin. The definiteness of the anatomical contours is partly an illusion. Each one of us is certainly far larger and more diffuse than his body."

- Plant physiologist Rupert Sheldrake in *A New Science of Life* postulated "morphogenetic fields" as invisible organizing fields which act across time and space and are responsible for forms and evolution, behavior and learning. Sheldrake concluded that, while neither mass nor energy, they "can be regarded as analogous to the known fields of physics in that they are capable of ordering physical changes, even though they themselves cannot be observed directly." His morphogenetic fields seem otherwise recognizable as aspects of the mental body, whether in an individual or in a group.

- Candace Pert, who performed groundbreaking research on neuropeptides at the National Institutes for Mental Health, reported in *Noetic Sciences Review* that "... it is possible now to conceive of mind and consciousness as an emanation of emotional information processing, and as such, mind and consciousness would appear to be independent of brain and body." She went on to say, "A mind is composed of information, and it has physical substrate that has to do with information flowing around. Perhaps, then, mind is the information among all these bodily parts. Maybe mind is what holds the network together."

One of the simplest ways to look at the brain-mind question (hinted at by Penfield above) and to arrive at a sense of the mind having "a life of its own" is by considering the sleep state. It takes little to recognize that during the hours of sleep, the mind allows the body to rest, much like computer operators do with their favorite device. The mind escapes the confines of the body and is active elsewhere. Just as the computer goes into a quiescent state when put to SLEEP, the body is in its own dormant condition when the mind- soul checks out for the night. Then, it flips back to active mode in the morning when the mind-soul makes its regular return.

Thus, we can visualize vital energy as the true skeleton of the human body and mind as the network which holds the whole being together. Just imagine for a moment what medicine will be like when these understandings are expanded and doctors carry such awareness into each clinic consult, hospital visit, and house call. Frugal Physicians already intuit this information so they can much more naturally lead their patients toward wholeness and healing.

True Psychology

Medicine ventured into psychology in the 19th century thanks to pioneering physicians. But with some exceptions, they followed patterns set by the orthodoxy. Early psychiatrists were trained in neurology (study of brain and nervous systems) and, to this day, most of their descendants look at mental problems as caused by faulty body physiology. Thus, the ready predilection to medicate their patients after surmising chemical imbalances. Even psychiatry is thus materialistic and body and brain based.

The mind certainly deserves more attention in medical school and medical practice. Real Physicians must be adept at psychology for a host of reasons. Here are just a few:
• Since the "body is in the mind," it falls prey to mental-emotional

problems in many ways. In fact, the body is clearly the slave of the mind. Many minds are unfocused, overly sensitive to surrounding minds and energies, and fogged by worries and fears which cannot but sooner or later influence the dependent body.

Being "in the mind," the body is subject to all kinds of mental stresses. Physicians need to read beyond symptoms to deeper layers in their patients' beings and lives.

• Varying figures suggest that 90 percent of illness is "stress related." While "stress related" often means "We Don't Know," it usually hints at emotional overlay, common anxiety, and simple inability to deal with the pressures of modern life. These develop differently depending on the individual.

One man's stress can be another man's pleasure. Some people thrive on high intensity, frequent change, and deadlines. They may well go 'stir crazy' when there is nothing to do. Sitting still can be like a death sentence for them. These folks might be considered Type A in recent terminology. Other behaviors are quite the opposite.

Physicians must recognize what kind of people they are consulting with. Similar symptoms in different patients can easily equate to fundamentally different dis-ease even though the presenting pictures may be much the same.

• Psychology is even more important in certain medical specialties. Can you guess which ones? A clue might help: Those who work with patients particularly subject to the influence by the minds and feelings of others.

Other people's minds influence all of us. But generally speaking, children and animals are at the low end of the totem pole in this part of life. If nought else, they often have limited ways to express and deal with what is going on inside of them. So, pediatricians and veterinarians have extra need of psychological skills.

Both children and animals have relatively undeveloped minds and can't help but be highly impressed by "larger" minds around them. Put differently, children and domesticated creatures can become overly influenced by the auras (mental-emotional fields) of family and owners. To their detriment in many cases. The older and the infirm may fit this picture as well.

Pediatricians need psychologic skills from the get-go because they have to go through parents and guardians in order to gather information. They quite often are treating parents more than children, whether they recognize it or not.

My pediatric experiences are limited. But, one episode comes to mind from days when I worked as a nurse at the Emergency Room of Fort Worth Osteopathic Hospital. A man in his late thirties came in with abdominal complaints. Prior to my calling for the physician, the patient ran over his medical history and pulled up his shirt to show me the three surgical scars he had on his abdomen. I couldn't help thinking that with just one more his family and friends could play tic-tac-toe on his belly. The man's influence on his seven-year-old son seemed quite obvious when the little boy pulled up his shirt to show off his own belly. No scars, yet!

Here is another sort of pediatric story drawn from a medical conference I attended many years ago. The speaker was an anthropologist who was working with the problem of obesity. He wanted us to know that that situation was not so strange because all sorts of disciplines had gotten involved in obesity with questionable results. An anthropologist might have new and useful insights.

His main premise was capsulized in a slide he projected on the big screen in front of us. It showed a very large man sitting in front of the television with both hands and mouth full of food. The next slide expanded on the first to show his equally obese wife doing pretty much the same thing. The punch line came in when young daughter and son, both chunky and overweight and chomping away, were added to the picture. But, the real kicker came when a fat cat and plump dog were shown in the full image on the last slide.

That animals are mentally affected by their owners should be a "no-brainer." But, all too often masters blame their relatively robotic cats and dogs when they act up. Or are totally nonplussed when their favorite pets get sick with illnesses much like their own.

The author is quite sure that domesticated animals loyally but unknowingly take on their owners' pain and emotional refuse and disease. They often make the ultimate sacrifice dying earlier than their time due to the ills unconsciously foisted upon them by their beloved masters.

- Perception is so very important in everyone's life. But most particularly in time of illness. If we think a problem is "big," it will surely become so whatever the physician tries to do.

Perceptions of physician are equally significant. Clouds of doubt and distress due to inharmonious physician-patient interactions can add hugely to the burdens of illness and the fears for the future that patients carry. This is another area of medical practice which has been largely ignored and needs to be addressed in future days.

In those times, medical schools will start from the "top down" to train students in mental sciences first and the physical ones later. As that occurs, psychology will also be much more prominent in all education and in child rearing. We will turn the old adage around to say, "A sound body in a sound mind."

Another layer of the human onion will eventually have to be peeled and this should naturally occur through the discipline of psychology. Our present psychological studies barely begin to hint at our deeper potentials and realities. What really sets humans apart from the crowd is their possession of individual souls.

Some day, psychology - the study of mind - most generally sick minds, will enter into its now esoteric work of uncovering the soul. Sad to say, medics have forgotten or given up finding the soul. Interesting, since that is our deepest and continuing nature.

But, psychology at least is on target by way of its name to open medicine and society to the idea of soul. Because its truest meaning is the study of the soul: psyche = soul, logy = study.

Scientists have had great difficulty coming to terms with the idea of mind. Most still believe it to be synonymous with brain. Humans with souls is even scarier to physically oriented physicians. "This reminds one of the story of the materialistic doctor who said he had done hundreds of post mortem examinations, but had never yet discovered the trace of the soul." (Arthur Avalon)

The soul is neither accessible to a surgeon's operation nor a pathologist's autopsy. But, Eastern yogis and teachers have known for centuries about the pathways for energies of the Soul into the mind and body.

"While, according to Western conceptions, the brain is the exclusive seat of consciousness, yogic experience shows that our brain-consciousness is only one among a number of possible forms of consciousness, and that these, according to their function and nature, can be localized or centered in various organs in the body." (Anagarika Govinda)

The midway or meeting point for these invisible forces and the outer physical human form is the psycho-neuro-endocrine system. The concept of this system is really quite simple while the practical explication of this subtle network will take long and inventive study. Direct support for this view is now coming from a new slowly evolving medical discipline called psycho-neuro-immunology. Psycho-neuro-immunology springs from the earlier arena of psycho-somatic medicine and will eventually form the scientific foundation of the inclusive field of psycho-neuro-endocrinology.

The following suggestions arise in the correlation of the components of a new psycho-physiological system starting with well known concepts from psycho-neuro-immunology:

1) The immune system is centered in the thymus gland located above the heart in the chest cavity.

2) The thymus gland is also one of the body's seven major human endocrine glands.

3) All of the glands, through their hormones which are secreted directly into the bloodstream, have profound effects upon the physical body.

4) The glands are interconnected and interrelated through feedback mechanisms, the master gland, and the nervous system.

5) The nervous apparatus and the endocrine glands actually make up one whole neuro-endocrine system.

6) The brain is the most important, but not the only nerve center, which influences the endocrine glands and the immune system.

7) The brain and other nerve centers and the endocrine glands are dependent upon emotions, the mind and the soul through the whole of the psycho-neuro-endocrine system.

The psychic (soul) end of the system is formed by the chakras (Sanskrit for wheel). They work through the mental and subtle bodies to manifest effects in brain and nerve centers, endocrine glands and bloodstream, organs and organ systems, body regions and parts towards illness or health. The psycho-physical energy centers (chakras) are constantly and progressively working to transmit the deeper, subtler, and most potent energies of creation into the human organism and into the human community. (See Appendix Illustrations.)

The united function of the nervous and endocrine systems has been hypothesized and demonstrated for many years in the West. "Hence in the largest sense the autonomic nervous system and the various endocrine glands (merged through the hypothalamus) represent a single neuroendocrine system that has evolved to integrate and coordinate the metabolic activities of the organism." (*Williams's Textbook of Endocrinology*) Although these systems are now separated by specialization in medical practice, this state assuredly will be modified in the future.

Eventually, body, mind and soul will be seen in life as the unified whole which they are. Thus creating a large picture upon which physicians and scientists can draw to produce an integrated and functional system of medicine and healing. In the meantime, Frugal Physicians use intuitive eyes and ears to relate to the ultimately whole patients they encounter.

Depth Physiology

Understanding of the psycho-neuro-endocrine system has practical implications for explaining a large portion of human ailments as they take us back to their true origins in the mental-emotional realms. Another portion of our ills arise simply from the way we humans process energy and the quality of those energies with which our bodies were built and are continually being rebuilt. Some illnesses involve a combination of these two factors.

The second set of problems relates to the simple idea that "Man does not live by bread alone." Certainly our bodies are affected by the kinds of food we consume and other things which they inhale and ingest in various ways. But, every thinking person must realize that while nutrition is important, it is only a small part of the story. This fact can be brought home by consideration of just a few examples:

• How many people do you know who manage to get the minimum daily requirements (MDRs) of vitamins and minerals every day? Teenagers who live for years on macaroni and cheese, twinkies and soda pop surely don't. Many hospital patients - especially when they don't eat their whole meals - don't. Many elderly people eat one meal a day, sometimes that being just a TV dinner. How is it possible for these folks to get the supposed necessary nutrients?

Even among so-called normal adults, it is questionable how many people eat optimally each day from the four basic food groups. Yet, most westerners are relatively healthy. At least relatively. Health is obviously dependent upon more than vitamins and minerals.

• Protein is the big concern for many people, including physicians, when vegetarian diets are begun. But, there seems to be little or no evidence that vegetarians - even vegans - become protein depleted following their dietary regimens.

Physicians, dietitians and nutritionists make recommendations for vegetarians to insure they get "complete proteins" by eating food combinations with all of the essential amino acids (protein building blocks). The author has been a vegetarian for most of his adult life, never concerned himself with such ideas, and has just as robust health as any meat-eater he has encountered. The general run of medical studies suggest that vegetarians are healthier on average than their carnivorous, protein-enriched brethren. Perfect protein intake is not required to live healthfully.

- Thousands of people go on fasts each year, generally they say for their betterment. Physicians don't get concerned on a fast of a few days. But when people - especially notables - go on political fasts or prisoners go on hunger strikes, medics get up in arms. Concerned that illness or even death might attend such acts. But, adverse effects from such actions are rare indeed.

Numerous famous "freedom fighters" have starved themselves for weeks, sometimes months, with only a certain amount of weight loss to show for their foodlessness. A number of saints of East and West are known to have lived for years with absolutely no food intake at all. Therese Neumann, mystic and stigmatist, consumed one eucharistic wafer a day as her only "food" for over 40 years.

Food appears to be optional for the health of some of our human kin. How about the rest of us? Maybe meals are just a habit.

- Yogis and fakirs of the East are known to have been entombed for weeks at a time without food, water, sunshine or air. When extracted from their cages, they generally appear no worse for the wear. These practices are not just limited to ancient times, but still go on among certain Indian ascetics.

Even in the West, we have self-proclaimed breatharians. Others say they live by gazing into the sun for certain times each day.

What makes these humans different? What do they know that we don't know such that they can live for extended periods without food and water and air and heat?

- The author's own limited outdoor experience suggests to him that all humans have natural capabilities similar to those noted above. But, these are little developed and little used, as we absorb regular meals, water intake, air flow and sunshine.

The writer has noticed that even with little sleep and food on camping ventures, he has felt more alive and invigorated than ever arising from a bed. A bed gives comfort, the elements give life. On a cross-country trek of five months, he lived quite well on liquids, granola bars and an occasional meal.

• There are numerous stories of people lost at sea, in the desert, and in the mountains who have survived well on little or no food for weeks at a time. Unfortunately, the "magic" of such incidents is often quickly forgotten in the elation of rescue and homecoming.

All of these anecdotes and stories give evidence - they do not prove - that humans have other "food sources" than the usual plant and animal kind. Traditions from the world round tell us that life- giving energies constantly surround us. They not only surround us but also pour into us and are our true food. Some of these energies are absorbed through food, others through breathing, and the rest through direct contact. The universe is a veritable waystation of multitudinous energies. We need never have fear of "running out of energy" when we begin to recognize and consciously use the vast networks and amazing flows of subtle energies which surround us at ALL times. (See Appendix Illustrations.)

These energies have long been known as the qi of the Chinese, prana of the Vedas, tLung of Tibet, aether of Greeks, od of Reichenbach and orgone of Reich, L-fields of Burr, etc. The list of names is long, entangled, and entirely in disrepute with most orthodox scientists who refuse to consider non-material concepts.

Science has battled with superstition in past centuries to maintain its total focus on the physical-material world. Still, the sciences must eventually - as physics has begun - rediscover "etheric" energies so as to fill gaps in so much of their work, to integrate the astronomical and the atomic, and to make sense of what really goes on within human beings.

Some day, scientists and physicians may merely sit back and

contemplate the nature of things - with mind, blackboard and chalk as Einstein did. They will inevitably be blessed with some "Aha!" moments and lift the blinders, open blank spaces in their limited thinking, and recover that which has been lost to them while still ever-present.

"There is nothing new under the Sun," so said a wise man of ancient times. The case is unchanged into our modern but only somewhat advanced times. Yet, all around us are unrecognized and unutilized forces.

The Scientific Revolution has barely scratched the surface. Though the natural worlds have revealed radiations and rays of many kinds, electricity and electronics, magnets and magnetism, atomic and nuclear energy. Grand as these discoveries have been, many more are yet to come forth when timid scientists dare look into places which to this point only the brave and wise, reckless and foolish have previously entered. These worlds will teach us about psychic healing, clairvoyance, telepathy, spiritualism, dowsing, mesmerism, animal magnetism, extra-sensory perception, karma and reincarnation.

The next steps taken will show the human body as an energy receiver, distributor and transmitter. Thus will a significant portion of human ills be explained by demonstrating that some bodies are prone to become congested with energy, others have blocks to reception, still others pass energy through at alarmingly fast rates, and still others are imbalanced in how they process and distribute within the body's own energy scheme.

ENERGY is such a BIG word at this time in history. Maybe that gives another sign that ENERGY will become BIG in medicine and healing as well as in so many other aspects of modern life.

Cause and Effect

Verlfying that subtle energies underlie the physical frame will form the first great step in understanding health and disease. Some day, this idea will be considered, "Elementary, my dear Watson."

The physical body and energy body are really both material in nature. One is very dense and relatively slow to change, the other fine and ever-moving and ever-changing. The latter qualities allow for sudden and immediate shifts in health states - for good or ill. They also help explain many previously unexplainables.

Even more will inevitably be explained as we move toward the other end of the spectrum. Where the deeper parts of the human organism dwell. And, where the largest portion of illnesses in modern times and societies develop.

Wise Physicians have long known that the mind is key to health and disease. Regular Physicians give nodding consent to the idea, yet trudge ahead devotedly pointed with singular interest on the dense body and physical symptoms. That myopic approach has been perpetuated for centuries now.

Still, patients have managed better in recent times with modern treatments which may appear sophisticated, but are often still downright crude. Moderns stand up better to pills and surgery because they are generally well tended, live in adequate housing, have regular incomes and hopes for the future.

Many writers inside and outside of medicine have spoken eloquently about how mind and body interact, how health is an inside job, and how there is in fact rhyme and reason to the passages of dis-ease, illness and injury which we all go through. None has been more on target than the sagacious Englishman, Edward Bach. Bach, physician, researcher, homeopath, and creator of the original flower remedies, who wrote like an ancient mage:

"The main reason for the failure of modern medical science is that it is dealing with results and not causes. For many centuries, the real nature of disease has been masked by materialism, and thus disease itself has been given every opportunity of extending its ravages, since it has not been attacked at its origin. The situation is like an enemy strongly fortified in hills, continually waging guerrilla warfare in the country around, while the people, ignoring the fortified garrison, content themselves with repairing the damaged houses and burying the dead, which are the result of the raids of the marauders. So, generally speaking, is the situation in medicine today; nothing more than the patching up of those attacked and the burying of those who are slain, without a thought being given to the real stronghold.

"Disease is in essence the result of conflict between Soul and Mind, and will never be eradicated except by spiritual and mental effort. Such efforts, if properly made with understanding as we shall see later, can cure and prevent disease by removing those basic factors which are its primary cause. No effort directed to the body alone can do more than superficially repair damage, and in this there is no cure, since the cause is still operative and may at any moment again demonstrate its presence in another form. In fact, in many cases apparent recovery is harmful, since it hides from the patient the true cause of his trouble, and in the satisfaction of apparently renewed health, the real factor, being unnoticed, may gain in strength. Contrast these cases with that of the patient who knows, or who is by some wise physician instructed in, the nature of the adverse spiritual or mental forces at work, the result of which has precipitated what we call disease in the physical body. If that patient directly attempts to neutralize those forces, health improves as soon as this is successfully begun, and when it is completed the disease will disappear. This is true healing by attacking the stronghold, the very base of suffering.

"Let it be briefly stated that disease, though apparently so cruel, is in itself beneficent and for our good and, if rightly interpreted, it will guide us to our essential faults. If properly treated, it will be the cause of the removal of those faults and leave us better and greater than before. Suffering is a corrective to point out a lesson which by other means we have failed to grasp, and never can be eradicated until that lesson is learnt. Let it also be known that in those who understand and are able to read the significance of premonitory symptoms, disease may be prevented before its onset or aborted in its earlier stages if the proper corrective spiritual and mental efforts be undertaken. Nor need any case despair, however severe, for the fact that the individual is still granted physical life indicates that the Soul who rules is not without hope." (*Heal Thyself*)

Many physicians and patients are content to believe that "Stuff happens!" That bacteria take over. That illness befalls us. That Satan must have had a hand in things. Illness is either an accident or the fault of an other. Power is ceded from the "victim" to the perpetrator. Known, unknown or just imagined.

But, "Nothing just happens." Disease is not anonymous. We just aren't investigating beyond the hard outer surface to find valid answers. When will we begin to develop eyes to see the obvious which has been staring us in the face for so long?

Dis-ease may not always be predictable or easy to understand, but it is certainly causational. Let's repeat that the majority - although certainly not all - of modern ills are the result of inner - mental-emotional - conflict. Further, these ills find their way into outer expression in the physical body by way of the psycho-neuro- endocrine system.

There are clues to be found along the way toward unraveling causation in practically all ailments. A very vitalizing and far- reaching lead in these investigations comes with the suggestion that, "all disease processes and syndromes, not only are psychosomatic in their form ... but also are symbolic of that process clinging to that which is obsolete for the nature and for the self." (Paul Solomon)

Ultimately, Wise and Frugal Physicians recognize that disease is not an unholy accident nor chaotic, neither an evil conception nor monstrous external hex but a picture of inner forces coming into play in the spirit, mind and body of an individual. (The same situation occurs in epidemics and contagious disease. Only the affected organism is larger, being a community, nation, continent or the whole world.)

Healing Times

The wise man of Ecclesiastes told us millennia ago of the ever recurring times and seasons of life - to tear down and build up, to rend and mend. His essential thoughts remain so poignant and poetic that they were put into verse and made into a classic hymn to the turbulent

60s. Undoubtedly, King Solomon had personal as well as national ills in mind when he composed his proverbs and axioms. Health and disease, life and death are all parts of the natural order of things both great and small.

Most human beings ignore the obvious, run from the inevitable, and employ physicians in efforts to annihilate pain, destroy disease, and bypass death. We are often like children trying to find ways to get out of doing mandatory homework and chores.

Few people - children and students, patients and physicians - handle change well. But, life is nothing but change. However slowly it may arise in the course of some cycles. And change eventually brings problems as well as progression.

Carl Jung, himself a wise physician, once said, "We do not solve our problems, we outgrow them." How often do physicians of any era consider illness and injury as problems to be outgrown? Physicians are trained to intervene and fix things. They rarely take time to consider them in context, watch them evolve, and view the wholesome outcome.

During college, I worked for a time on weekends as an assistant to a hospital Xray technician. It was quite instructive to recognize how medical facilities keep the "revolving door" open for many patients. One particular weekend, an old fellow with a number of chronic problems appeared for his latest admission chest Xray.

I wheeled the patient into the "shooting room," listening to the banter between technician and patient. The two recognized each other from earlier trips to XRAY. The patient had been hospitalized in recent weeks. The tech, trying to be friendly, asked the man how he was doing. He replied, "Not so good or I wouldn't be here."

The technician picked up the thread of the conversation with all good intent and another kindly but not too wise thought, "Oh, you'll be okay. We'll have you back to your old self in no time."

I have heard that line numerous times over the years. But, that first incident stands out in my memory. I believe it suggests a valuable lesson for us. One part of the problem in much illness and trauma is simply the struggle involved in moving from the old self to the new self. This idea fits well with those of Dr. Bach (previous chapter) who would surely suggest that we are continually being drawn towards growth and transformation, the new self - or quite possibly the Self.

This state is often hard to recognize - very hard - when we are in pain, discomfort, confusion and fear. Nonetheless, there are times and seasons for disease and healing. As well as rhyme and reason to them. Physicians and patients need to learn to take the long view, look from the wide angle, and take in the whole panorama at the same time. It is possible, but it does take practice.

I had the occasion over the winter of 1995 to be a "consultant" with a friend and her family as she went through the early stages of a serious dis-ease. For several months, I actually became part of "the family." Karen's family. I call her Karen, because she was always "carin'" for others, most notably her husband and children. Karen and the Crabtree family lived in the Far West outside a small town populated with many granola folks and tree huggers. They topped the heap, more or less. Karen's husband, Herb, was a physician, tall and blond, sensitive, gentle, soft spoken, who had a small holistically oriented office in town. Karen had been a counselor until her three children arrived. She raised them, took care of the household, helped with the book work at the office, and recently had found time to get back to some of her counseling work. The three young people - teenagers on the way to adulthood were bright, talented, and energetic.

The whole family was as health oriented as one could imagine. They were vegetarian, mostly organic. No salt, little sugar. The youngest child wouldn't eat dairy products, but he made exceptions for ice cream.

The Crabtrees were into all sorts of exercise and outdoor activities - jogging, skiing, hiking, camping, swimming, cycling. Most of the family was musical and friends would be corralled on occasion for social nights including singing, instrumentals, stories and jokes. Early morning and late evening walks among the pine hills were also favorite pastimes for the family.

The whole "family" situation was idyllic. How could anything mar the life that the Crabtrees had built over 20 years?

But, the fairy tale began to unravel suddenly when Karen started to have seizures. Quickly, she was seen in a large medical center, scanned and diagnosed with a slow-growing but still inoperable brain tumor.

The good news was that the tumor was benign. The bad news came with the slow-growing part within the confines of the skull which might eventually squeeze the brain more severely than to just produce occasional fits. "It might have been developing for several years," she was told by a neurosurgeon who would not operate. At least, he wouldn't at that point in time. Other opinions were mixed, but no surgeon was eager to recommend surgery. The professional hope was that the tumor would grow very slowly to allow her to live to her old age. The seizures might be her only symptoms. And they might be controllable.

Those pronouncements sent Karen back to her own resources, alternatives, and inner guidance. Karen was a tall woman, sandy haired, soft and sensitive, always chipper and supportive of others. A real caregiver who may have been given an opportunity to be on the receiving end of things. But, Karen was used to being the giver and habits, even good ones, are hard to change.

With some family input, Karen decided to use a number of modalities including vitamins, visualization, art, exercise, and journaling to deal with her inoperable, slow-growing brain tumor. She also went to Episcopal prayer and healing services, consulted readers and took an occasional few days in southern California with her mother. But, being on her own away from her family was outside her comfort zone.

When I came into the picture a few weeks after the diagnosis, Karen and I got together once a week for some hands-on work and conversation. Becoming part of the family and one of her therapists, I was privileged to hear her recite snippets from the journal that she had begun to keep. She wrote religiously and voluminously filling one notebook after another every few weeks.

Karen took up the Ira Progoff method of journaling. As I understand, the journaler gets into a relaxed state of mind and addresses anything or anyone she wishes. Starts a give and take conversation. Karen did that and her most frequent conversationalist was her tumor.

I got to read some of the journaling that most captured her

attention. Ones that she thought worth sharing. The gist of the confabs seemed to come down to Karen's understandable fears and worries, and the tumor's efforts to explain that it had not come to destroy her but rather to change her life. Which it was surely doing, although maybe not always as intended.

Listening in, I couldn't help adding my take that the tumor was bringing her an opportunity instead of a problem. We - Karen and you and I - are so often, and sometimes easily, intimidated by our illnesses, that we miss out on their potential benefits. I repeated more than a few times in various ways that I believed, "This is meant to be a life-enhancing not life-threatening experience. Tumors are also called growths. This presence is benign and wants you to GROW, Karen."

Nevertheless, Karen focused on relieving herself, getting rid of the tumor which tried to insinuate to her that it was her friend. That was clearly hard for her to accept, but she kept talking and journaling. The simplest, most dramatic and eye-opening journaling conversation she ever shared with me was one that went like this:

Karen: When you go away, will I be healed?
Tumor: When you are healed, I will go away!
Bob: Wow!

The Gift of Disease

Human beings, physicians included, are very short sighted.

- We don't learn from the past. The words of Santayana, "Those who do cannot remember the past are condemned to repeat it," seem to have been meant for leaders of nations, but most assuredly fits individuals as well.

Much of disease clearly develops out of old patterns which we fail to outgrow. Old habits of acting, feeling, and thinking. It doesn't take a genius to recognize that we constantly build our tomorrows by how we live today. Illness and dis-ease should come as no real surprise to those with eyes open. If so, we should be able to prevent or mitigate much of it.

- We don't see the writing on the wall. We don't read the signs and symbols which are all around and within us, ever available to teach and guide us onward. The universe is continually giving us hints of what is coming.

Some say, "Your car is a sex symbol." But, there are many other signs along the way. Our homes and mates, friends and enemies, jobs and pastimes, failures and successes symbolize layers of our beings - problems and possibilities. So do our ailments and injuries.

- We get lost in the details and minutiae of life and ignore the essentials. We live in a magical, miraculous, mystical forest, so to speak, and we miss it because we spend so much of our time focused on one clump of trees, or a single sapling.

And then, we don't recognize the wholeness of that tree. We are oblivious to the fact that a large portion of tree matter is under ground. Even more of it extends above and below, within and around through its aura. We don't have to touch a tree to hug it.

Bringing the picture back to personal territory, humans focus on the outer ring of things rather than the inner core. We pay homage to the body - a fleeting thing - instead of the persisting soul.

- We are blind to reality and get entangled in superficial, transient dramas and traumas. We have small gods, think this one bodily excursion is it, have limited attention spans being captured in the day, and believe the world revolves around us.

Perspective, whether in health or disease, can make a huge difference in how our lives unfold and how we manage the apparent vagaries of existence.

Disease is never accidental. Cause and effect reign in all of our lives and even in the midst of illness, discord and disaster. To believe otherwise is really rather ludicrous and flies in the face of the grand order on which all things are created and sustained. It is near time for all of us to tune in, get with it, pick up the clues, and put them to good use for the betterment of all. In the meantime, "The Fates lead the willing, and drag the unwilling." (Seneca)

I wish I could say that my friend Karen read the clues and got the messages that the tumor was trying to share with her. Maybe she got some of them. I only read a few of her journal entries and only lived nearby for a few months before I returned to my mountain home. Nor could I or anyone know all the ramifications of things which go on in someone else's life. It is hard enough for us - even with our eyes open - to understand what is passing through our very own selves.

That said, this is how I remember the rest of the story. "Being healed" was the simple but elusive answer. The common thought is that health is the absence of disease. Karen thought if she could get the tumor to depart, she would be healed. The tumor suggested the opposite.

Still, she persisted focusing on the tumor. She worked on one of the in-things at the time, guided imagery and visualization. Karen added to her regimen sessions of visualizing her white blood cells in armies coming to - lovingly - detach tumors cells and carry them away to be flushed out of the body. Karen didn't want any violence done to the tiny cells. But, her focus was narrow. She still pointed mostly at her body and "getting rid of her tumor."

In our latter sessions together, I tried to get her involved in the idea of wholeness. Expanding her horizons outside of her family where she thought she was indispensable. Getting away for herself regularly. Letting her husband, children and friends live their lives and be responsible for themselves. So everyone could grow up.

I am reminded that Karen was a bit on the obsessive side. About some things, anyway, most particularly her family. Karen was one of only two people I ever met who arranged the wastebasket. The other was my former wife.

I endeavored to get Karen to understand that real healing resulted in wholeness. I didn't get too far. But, I was heartened on the day of my leaving the family and the area when Karen asked if I had any parting suggestions for her. I said, "No. But, I do have a question for you."

Bob: "What or who will you be when you are healed?"
Karen: "Oh, I will be an artist."
Bob: "How much time will you spend painting to get there?"
Karen: "Lots."

Would that had been the case. Another part of the story was that in years past - possibly coincident with the onset of the growth in her head - Karen had walked through a craft fair. Stopping at a particular stall, she became captivated by the pieces of water color art on display. She broke down in tears, thinking, "Oh, that is wonderful. I should paint like that. I can do that. I must."

Karen had taken art classes intermittently over intervening years and became a credible artist. But, she never thought she was good enough. Always needing to take more classes. Keeping only a small corner in her bedroom for her work and never making it a priority. Even after declaring, "I will be an artist."

For a fleeting moment, however, she permitted some of her pieces to be sold on auction at a benefit done for her. She then made some other pieces into greetings cards and began to open the door to become that artist.

After I left, we communicated regularly for a time and then less so. Later, I received updates from her sister. The story seemed to be that Karen couldn't push herself to "Be an artist." Family and other obligations came first. She didn't take much time away from home "responsibilities" either to explore the world and her talents or even to invest in her deeper self.

By the time I saw Karen again - seven years later - on a brief visit to "the family," she had undergone two surgeries for her supposed "inoperable tumor" as well as other aggressive treatment. Two of her three children were in college. The third was in his final year of high school.

Her husband had found another woman, and Karen and Herb were divorced. Karen was alone except for her son who would soon be gone.

Her artistic dreams had slipped away, the tumor remained and continued to grow despite de-bulking surgeries. Karen had not been healed yet. Else the tumor would have gone of its own accord. Even at that visit, Karen was nearing death's door. She got around with help and talked a bit. Mrs. Crabtree joined the family including her then former husband for Thanksgiving dinner in a sad moment. Karen died a few weeks later. Where the growth then took her I cannot say. But assuredly into deeper levels of healing.

The Patients of Job

In a perfect world, the onset of disease and the event of injury will be looked upon as opportunities for learning. Rather than times to take up defensive positions, prepare battle lines, and call in the reinforcements.

Fighting disease is far and wide the most common approach. Few patients recognize the potential gifts offered them. The mindset and training of physicians and patients will change, but slowly. This is largely because systems keep the prevailing aggressive medical perspective armed and in power. Disease is IN.

I am reminded of another world depicted by Samuel Butler in his book Erewhon. Erewhon is an anagram for the word nowhere. The central character finds himself unexpectedly in a distant country where things clearly run at odds to the "real world" he is used to. Most pertinently, insane people are coddled and the physically sick are treated like criminals.

Similarly, our own world seems to have things backwards with regard to illness and therapy. Physicians and patients miss out on the opportunities that disease present because:

• we are most often in a hurry to feel better, return to normal, and recover the old self. All such actions should be subject to review.
• we don't like being ill. Clearly, illness is deemed abnormal and unacceptable. Not part of the plan. But, then as the saying goes, "Life

happens while we are making plans."
- we need permission to be ill. From ourselves and our many responsibilities, our employers and schools, the insurance company, and our usual way of living.
- the system only gives us permission to be sick or absent for a few days each year.
- medical doctors are often required to authenticate and to authorize "genuine" disease.

The writer has come to the conclusion that changing this part of medicine and healing will necessitate physicians taking time to ponder and seek to understand their own illnesses and injuries. Medical schools are generally happy to matriculate students who have had hospital and clinical experience of one kind or another. But, it will be a hard sell for medical schools to require prospective medical students to have had some "experience" of prolonged illness, medical intervention, and hospitalization. Still, we might wonder how the experiences of illness or injury and patienthood would change the way the medical system works.

At one time while working in later years in a hospital education department, my supervisor and I studied the idea of presenting the film, *The Doctor*, as an opportunity for workers - hopefully to include physicians - to take another look at the experience of illness. The effort never came to fruition and may not have been accepted well if accomplished. The common resistance among doctors to new ideas was always in mind as we considered our eventually aborted project.

Based on Dr. Edward Rosenbaum's book *A Taste of My Own Medicine: When The Doctor Is The Patient*, the film tells about a successful, talented cardio-thoracic surgeon who has no bedside manner, is bent on getting as much work out of each day and his staff as possible, and has a "get-in, get-out, get-it-over" attitude. But, The Doctor eventually Gets It himself.

Driving home with his wife from a professional dinner, Dr. Jack MacKee has a fit of coughing up bright red blood on the interior of their new car. The frustrating demeaning experience of having a biopsy done by an insensitive specialist follows as does diagnosis of throat cancer.

Jack encounters cold and emotionally sterile hospitals with physicians to match. He begins to empathize with patients and recognize the kind of medic he used to be. MacKee befriends a cancer patient with an inoperable brain tumor who eventually dies.

Jack recovers and is changed dramatically. When he returns to work, he begins to teach interns compassion and sensitivity towards their patients. He also gives them opportunities to learn what is like to be on the other side of the stethoscope by making his residents and interns "become patients" and be treated so in the hospital for a few days.

It is not clear that *The Doctor* ever learned patience, but he certainly slowed down. The writer has had his own encounters with dis-ease which have helped him learn patience with the processes of life, recognize that he is often not in charge of his own body, and that time is one of the great healers. Both physicians and patients hopefully will also gain more of these understandings in the future.

Put very simply: "Patients need patience."

There are many ways to learn as well as different kinds of learners. But, most will agree that learning by doing is a superior method. There is plenty of that in medical training, especially in later years. "Learning by being (a patient)" has yet to make advances into the system.

It generally only happens later in life for physicians. Even then, physicians often are treated with "professional courtesy" and are rewarded for being part of the "medical club." So, they may miss out on many possible learning opportunities. Still, disease by itself - regardless of medical care - can be a potent and lasting teacher.

The author has been fortunate as far as health goes. He has a relatively high pain threshold and has experienced very few ills before wearing the cap and gown of a medical school graduate. His bodily misfortunes have been limited to minor injuries, tonsillitis, colds and "sinus infections," one bout of hepatitis, and car karma. At least that was the case until the Big One hit.

It was midwinter 2001 in Montana, a mild one as is common. That Montana winters are often so is a guarded secret. I was planning a long walk in the summer to New York City, intending to get things in order in the spring for a June departure.

By that time in my life, I had adopted a logo of sorts for myself: an American flag with but one star in the blue canton and that star covered partially by a golden heart. I first painted the emblem to cover a huge second story wall of The Rocky Mountain Garage, an old county garage which became the site of Red White and Blue Celebrations and other events in Lavina, Montana.

The symbol later became the focus of a quilt which was used as a backdrop for stage performances at the Garage. Eventually, it appeared as a machine-sewn nylon flag which I carried on my walk across the country. Interestingly with each new iteration of the logo, the heart got progressively larger until it bulged out beyond the limits of the star.

In early February out of the blue, I began having a diffuse, nagging heaviness in my chest. There was no pain. And no other symptoms. But, it gnawed and gnawed on me.

The focus of the discomfort began on the right side of my chest and slowly expanded to the whole region. It wouldn't go away regardless of what I did or didn't do. If I rested it was present. If I worked, it was still there. It didn't interfere with activity, but it was like a big sore thumb of which I was always aware.

The only "therapies" I used were rest, work, and hot baths. For many years, my habit has been to "tough out" practically all ailments and injuries that have become my lot. I have been fortunate to have a thick hide. I also have had jobs and living situations which allowed me to rest, recuperate and let nature "do its work" when I became ill or injured.

The heaviness and discomfort persisted. The only other problem which crept into my awareness was a growing sense of unease when around groups or crowds of people. I felt things closing in on me. It was a good time to be outside because the air and space made me a little more comfortable. Just going to the local cafe was sometimes a problem. Making trips into the Big City and visiting Walmart was sometimes really distressing.

Spring arrived and I was no better, but I got focused on Easter.

Reading stories from the Bible and other texts, I convinced myself that I was going to be "resurrected" from my ills with Easter.

Nothing happened until Sunday when I was invited to the home of the Browns to join in an Easter get-together and meal. The claustrophobic feeling soon appeared, I couldn't eat, I became afraid that I would pass out and fall into the food. Worse than that, I eventually thought, "I'm gonna die." It was a horrible, scary, no good, very bad feeling.

I got up from the table with the intention of walking home, but I only got as far as the couch. The Browns and the Hortons came to my rescue trying to help. "What can we do?" they asked, while Phil gave me a nitroglycerine tablet. I cooperated and took it.

"Call Ginger." Ginger was my significant other, at the time visiting her family in New York. Mrs. Brown got Ginger on the phone. I asked her to come back and sit with me. If I was going to die, I didn't want to be alone.

Ginger checked with the airlines. To get her ticket changed without extra cost required a physician's report. (It probably would have been cheaper to pay the extra fare instead of going through a medical consultation.) For the first time in twenty years, I took myself to a physician. Actually, Mrs. Brown drove me to the small hospital clinic in the next town.

The foreign-born physician with whom I consulted was both attentive and accommodating. I told him my story. He did a quick exam and suggested blood tests and an EKG. I asked him what he might find in blood work. We settled on an EKG which was "normal." Everything was "normal," except how I was feeling. The doctor recommended having a stress test at a cardiology clinic in the Big City. I thanked him and left with a note for the airlines.

I wasn't about to go near the Big City hospital. No telling what they might find or imagine me having. No knives, please. Besides, I had no insurance and was paying out of my pocket.

Synchronistically, my father back home in South Dakota was having his own chest problem. Months earlier, his physician had told him, "You probably have a hiatal hernia. Try these pills. Come back if you have need."

Well, he had need. My 89-year-old father had progressive symptoms. At almost exactly the same time I was having my Easter ills, Dad's problems got worse and he then was admitted to the local hospital. He had fluid in his chest which the medics drained.

My brother called and told me about my father. Despite my own ills, I decided I needed to go help out. I didn't feel up to driving 650 miles, so I intended to take the bus. But, that didn't seem to be a much better choice. Ginger volunteered to take me home. I slept in the back of her van during much of the trip.

We pulled into the hometown just as my brother arrived at my father's apartment house with Dad in tow following his discharge from the hospital. Ginger stayed a day or two while I took up residence as chief caregiver.

It was clear by then that my father had cancer and was entering his last days. Nonetheless, we had to go through the motions and take him to appointments as well as to another hospital admission for biopsy which unsurprisingly showed a malignant lung tumor.

My own discomfort was little changed wherever I was except again in crowds and inside the clinic and hospital. I recall helping my father stay upright while he had another chest Xray at the clinic. I feared that I might pass out and get run over to the Emergency Room with scary results.

I was with my father during all but a few hours of the last five weeks of his life. It was a trying but somehow magical experience. Strangely it took 52 years for me to realize how similar father and son were. I cared for him like a parent cares for a child. Fed him, bathed him, shaved him.

Along with Dad's chest problem, he developed weakness and diminished feeling in his legs. So, it was difficult for him to navigate. When he needed to move from one place to another, I gave him a hand and an arm, and we "danced across the room."

Eventually, he stopped eating and went to sleep for most of three days. He died in his favorite easy chair. His body was buried with military rites at the town cemetery next to mother's after a church service where the sons and family members and friends spoke in remembrance of him.

Ginger returned for the funeral and drove me back to Montana. By then, I was a bit better. Unexpectedly just a fortnight after Dad died, my chest discomfort disappeared. It had moved and been transformed into pain in my right hip. The problem had traveled a path like a figure 7 as it passed very, very slowly through my body. However uncomfortable the hip pain was, I was relieved and quite thankful. "I'm not gonna die."

While the chest problem lasted four months, the hip pain covered five more. Then, voila! Both were gone. No worse for the wear. But, I wouldn't want to go through it again. No siree, Bob.

Nine months. It had been like giving birth. Seemingly to the new me. One who was able a year past schedule to walk across the country. I must admit that I did have some trouble for a few weeks getting used to a backpack while preparing for the trip. Even an unweighted pack was more than I could bear. But slowly, that unease dissipated and I was good to go on June 11, 2002, for a five month journey across America.

To this point in my life, I consider the two experiences recounted above as the most important of my career. Five weeks tending my father in his last days. And five months walking across the great American land. The two helped expand my heart and make me ready for further steps on the path of life. Being reminded of walking miles and miles and miles brings up the old Native American metaphor: "You can't really understand another man until you live his life, walk in his shoes." Such a thing is very hard to do. But, it is something a Frugal Physician really ought to ponder on. Especially if s/he has never had a significant medical problem. And then again, even if s/he has.

Going the Distance

We so commonly and readily think of our down times, hurts and pains, discomforts and dis-ease as bad, harmful and evil. How limited that view is like many others typical to modern humans. We have - as a race - lost touch with or have yet to recognize -

    the wonder of nature   the gift of disease
    the magic of life   the challenge of growth
    the hidden worlds within   the everpresent spirit
    the amazing cycles of birth and life, death and rebirth

The wondrous thing about life is that even when we endeavor to avoid the teachings of illness and injury, they will most certainly continue to follow us. Our ultimate choice is not whether we will be taught but how long it will take us to learn.

"A rich and mighty Persian once walked in his garden with one of his servants. The servant cried that he had just encountered Death, who had threatened him. He begged his master to give him his fastest horse so that he could make haste and flee to Teheran, which he could reach that same evening. The master consented and the servant galloped off on the horse. On returning to his house the master himself met Death, and questioned him, 'Why did you terrify and threaten my servant?' 'I did not threaten him; I only showed surprise in still finding him here when I planned to meet him tonight in Teheran,' said Death." (Viktor Frankl)

Viktor Frankl's story can be used for many purposes. It fits with the old adage: "You can run but you can't hide." You can run but you can't hide from what dis-ease is trying to teach. Fortunately, its teachings ultimately work for good. Even when clumsy technicians, insensitive practitioners, and sterile hospitals intervene.

I have had the chance to see this demonstrated in many cases. My only wonderment has been, "Why does it have to be so hard and brutal and caustic and bloody?" I have wondered more than a few times whether medical practitioners and hospitals in the modern era somehow substitute for the tormentors and torturers of ages past. They too used poisons and blades, extracted blood and gave electric shocks. It seems that modern medics unconsciously create extraordinary experiences for their patients which even ancient inquisitors may have never dreamed of.

This situation happens so frequently in the treatment of cancer that every reader must know some friend or family member who has submitted to such well-meaning but sadly disturbing therapies. While the causes of cancer are almost totally unknown, medical people still persist with their violent ways in poisoning (chemo), burning (radiation), and cutting (surgery) in search of cure.

Strangely, medical exorcism seems to work in a portion of those who submit. But is it because:

- the treatment is correct?
- the patient's will to live is stronger than disease AND treatment?
- the patient's soul decides it is not time to leave the body?
- the disease and/or treatment are necessary to patient growth?

The author believes that in the large majority of cases the last three reasons cover the territory well. Putting these three together suggests that for many patients these sorts of travails are part of the pathway to the new self. A pathway which cannot be found in the present day as it was in past times.

- For ages, human beings were stressed and stretched by living close to the elements. They lived very close to earth, water, fire and air which provided contact with energies which modern westerners can hardly even imagine.

- Rites of passage were part of the norm in bygone days. Men and women went through them at different times in their lives to prove themselves, "earn their spurs," make the grade. In the present day, a relative few in the military go through such testing.

- Testing in combat was so common until recent times. Practically every generation saw men go off to battle. Thousands and millions were tried under fire - literally and figuratively.

- The medicine men of primitive groups had to endure major illness and trials, passing through altered states so that they might deserve their lot as leaders. Vision quests, sacred dances, and ceremonials also had their place in the process.

For many moderns, the medical experience can take the place of trials with the elements, rites of passage, military fire, and initiation. Many of the cancer patients I have worked with were shocked or drugged into states of consciousness that they had no other way of experiencing. Just being anesthetized certainly disconnects patients from body and brain, and takes them into other worlds. Worlds perhaps where real healing is more possible or likely.

I remember staring at leukemic patients who had had the blood practically drained from their vessels, hair lost, body emaciated. They were placed in - to outward view - a state of limbo, awaiting some inner transformation. Such treatment can't help but "rattle a person's cage." Which metaphor might be apt.

Years ago, a 19-year-old neighbor friend developed leukemia. I visited him in the hospital through his ordeal. He was a busboy and a slow learner. His family had no money. There was no telling how he paid his medical bill. Out of his struggle, the young man became a bit of a celebrity for a time. He survived leukemia and his treatment. He went on to college and a previously unexpected life.

"Contemporary man ... is blind to the fact that, with all his rationality and efficiency, he is possessed by 'powers' that are beyond his control. His gods and demons have not disappeared at all; they have merely got new names. They keep him on the run with restlessness, vague apprehensions, psychological complications, an insatiable need for pills, alcohol, tobacco, food -- and, above all, a large array of neuroses." (Carl Jung)

Everyday illness and injury must be added to Dr. Jung's list. They are often the result of unhonored powers within. We have advanced little over the centuries, continuing as we do to deal with our inner conflicts in often painful and unconscious ways. That our problems find their ways into our bodies is not to be denied. That they must be addressed with modern crudities which are akin to purging, bleeding and leeching is hard to fathom.

Enlightened ancients took themselves to healing temples where they may have been medically treated but also incubated as if infants. Placed in quiet spaces, prompted to dream, to "visit inner worlds," to commune with oracles, to be touched by the Wise Ones. Frugal Physicians of the future must resurrect a semblance of those times and those methods. We must recall those moments when the body was understood as the outer garment of mental-emotional

beings on the path to integration and healing with their souls.

Temples of Healing

Hospitals and clinics have become centers of all kinds of activities. Healing occasionally occurs in those institutions but it is not all that common due to many of the reasons which have been discussed in the preceding chapters.

To our detriment as whole people and whole societies, medicine and healing have been expropriated from the public. Medicine has practically led the way in separating key parts of human life away from home, family and community. This has not been done meanly and often not even intentionally. But over time "for your own good," much like the many well-meaning, but misguided efforts of caring governments.

Specialization and technology, legalisms and "progress" have separated birth and death, illness and injury from their natural habitat. Huge hospital temples and clinic consortiums as well as smaller versions have extracted much of human experience from their natural settings and placed them in dull, cold boxes. Where professionals deliver out one-size-fits-all service.

Medical attempts at healing have become mercenary practices. We pay people to fix us, take care of our problems, and relieve us of the ill effects of our lifestyles and habits, karma and aging. That practice is not unlike our volunteer, mercenary military. Rather than fight our own battles, we pay the young, the poor, and the dark-skinned to defend our nation. "Die for us, if you must."

Physicians aren't about to die for us, but they certainly will try to stand between us and our problems by focusing them onto our physical bodies. Then, they fight phantom enemies for us.

Still, physicians are ultimately not the problem. We are the problem. We have allowed the management of health and healing, disease and death to go far astray. It is the whole society which has been carried out onto a limb. It is long past time for:

- people to address their own health problems.
- families to assert themselves as caregivers.
- the public to study their bodies, health, and lives.
- the facts of subtle energies to become commonly known.
- the wonders of life itself to animate our communities.

Dramatic changes in the future are not going to come simply via more specialization, enhanced technologies, and even Frugal Physicians. They will arise when individuals begin to take more responsibility for themselves and neighbors, and when communities become temples of healing again.

All sectors and disciplines in the society - including education, law, and religion - must resume their parts in the health equation. That may cause some real battles over turf. But, health is not just a medical concern. It is a universal one, albeit with unique aspects in the western world.

Mother Teresa of India has oft been quoted as saying, "The problem of the East is material deprivation. The problem of the West is spiritual deprivation." Viewing life from that angle, it may be of some advantage to be poor in India or in the United States.

Less medical care may be better for you. You won't have your pockets picked so readily. You won't be overmedicated. You won't have needless and dangerous procedures done upon your body. You won't be diagnosed with non-existent diseases. You may still be uncomfortable, but you will have your own problems as well as opportunities to learn from them.

If you are poor, you will be more likely to ask for help from parents, siblings, kin, and neighbors as in third world countries. You may be willing to knock on the door of the neighborhood elder. You may not feel stupid when you ask your grandmother about home remedies. You may be happy to call for your neighbor's assistance in later years rather than submit to nursing home services. Psychiatrist M. Scott Peck has said in his book *A Different Drum,*

"The pathway to salvation in the modern world is through community." I think that he might have been willing to include healing under the label "salvation." Community is hardly the whole answer because we all have to take some responsibility for ourselves, but it surely is something that has been lost to moderns in recent generations and needs to be redeveloped.

Numerous stories come to mind which address the idea of community involvement in healing. We all can recite how our towns and cities have added to illness and injury, but there are many ways for real community to make differences in the opposite direction.

It seems to be in vogue now for groups to get together to raise money to fight or defeat this disease or the other, to produce a benefit for sufferers of disease or accident, and to dramatize colorfully and actively some quasi-medical organization. Most of these endeavors are well intentioned and produce good feelings. But, they also keep money rolling into the medical system and building more monuments to Cancer, Muscular Dystrophy, Multiple Sclerosis, etc. Job security has been relatively unchallenged in such organizations for a long time. While cures have been few, the charities have gotten larger and larger. A friend reminds me that, "Doctors have garnered much more money than cures from cancer treatment." Communities need to be mobilized for self healing, not merely to promote expensive causes and bigger medicine.

Some vignettes follow on the problems and possibilities which surround the idea of community healing.

• There must have been a better way, but . . . My brother and his wife were going through bankruptcy many years ago in my home town. My octogenarian father and equally old maternal aunt were the only close relatives in the vicinity. Still, there were some cousins nearby and neighbors and their church.

My sister-in-law became acutely ill. Diagnosed with pneumonia, she was prescribed medication, time off from school teaching, and strict bed rest. The latter seemed unlikely because of three young children in the house. She submitted to being hospitalized instead of going home.

This incident might well have been a perfect opportunity for community support and healing, from more than just one angle. Instead, the hospital became an expensive - to the insurance company - place of rest and respite. Healing? That was questionable because the stress of bankruptcy continued for many months.

• Healing can happen anywhere and does. If "Anything can cure anything," then healing can happen most anywhere. And, it surely happens more often anywhere than in medical facilities. Think about it.

During my medical practice years, I frequented workshops on holistic medicine and spirituality which caught my attention and fit my budget and schedule. One of my fondest memories is that of experiencing the talents of a man named Jim Turner.

Turner was a musician from the Rockies who created music using all sorts of unusual implements: baking pans, wine glasses, wrenches and handsaws to name a few. He was good enough to catch Johnny Carson's attention and appear on the Tonight Show. He apparently has given up that business because internet searches for him turn up empty. Maybe he went into healing work. He had the knack.

While performing a number of songs on his Sandvig handsaw at a medical convention, he told about playing some of the same numbers on a recent return visit to a church in Colorado. At the end of that show, he shook hands with members of the audience who passed through a receiving line. An older woman got his attention and initiated a conversation. She told him, "The last time you played here, you gave me a bloody nose."

Turner was a little embarrassed and at a loss as to what to say, so he tried to apologize. The woman stopped him and said, "Oh, no. It was really wonderful what happened that night."

The lady related how she had grown up in a family in which expression of feelings was not allowed. She married a man who was much the same. So, she continued to hold things in even after her husband died. In later years, she developed high blood pressure which was not well controlled on medication. Her physician told her he was worried.

Turner's first musical performance enthralled the woman. When he played *Jesu, Joy of Man's Desiring* on his saw, she couldn't hold her feelings back any longer. They broke through, not in tears but in a bloody nose. Her physician then told her he had been worried that her unrelieved blood pressure might some day result in a stroke. He was then pleased and hopeful because of the change that happened on her experiencing Jim Turner's touching music.

With several hundred in an amphitheater setting, Mr. Turner concluded his evening session conducting the group as a glass harmonica orchestra. Everyone got a wine glass. Different sections had glasses with different amounts of water in them. As Jim played his handsaw, he pointed groups to join in and drop out. All we did was wet our fingers and rub the rims of the glasses, each section producing its own wonderful tone to add to the unique symphony.

The music was ethereal and the event truly memorable. Thanks, Jim, for that magical moment of healing.

• Years ago I led a workshop on Spiritual Healing in which I asked participants to get into groups and discuss one quotation from a list I provided which spoke to the idea of "mind as builder." Each group was to consider their chosen quote plus another which simply stated: "Jesus Christ was a carpenter." There was one quotation which remained unchosen and I decided to work on it while the groups conferred.

A young man came forward and said that he wanted to join me. The odd quote was rather deep and we didn't get far with it. But when we considered the idea that "Jesus Christ was a carpenter," we did much better. My partner, Sid, shared that he was a professional carpenter. He volunteered how a carpenter uses tools and materials to create something new and valuable. He then suggested how Christ was working even then to build us into new and better beings.

His words were so clear and poignant that I asked him to share with the larger group (about 80 people) when we got back together. Sid resisted doggedly. He was really quite shy, afraid to speak in front of a crowd and avoided such at all costs, he told me. But, I "dogged" him and gave him the choice of talking from his chair in the audience or standing with me up front to tell his thoughts.

Sid didn't like the choices, but he eventually stood up next to his woman friend, Ms. Carpenter, and made a little speech using the ideas he had shared with me. The audience applauded and I offered that the group had just witnessed an effort at building wholeness and a moment of healing.

- An apochryphal story is retold of an ancient Essene healing community which existed along the River Jordan. The Master Jesus was said to spend time there. His presence drew many visitors and instantaneous healings occurred on occasion like those recorded in the New Testament. Most generally, healing was a process, rather than an event, which involved caring over long periods for the ill and needy.

Physicians traveled from great distances hoping to discover the latest "technology," learn the secrets of the Master, and be inspired and rejuvenated in their own healing works. Some went away disappointed because "Miracles" were few and far between.

Still, there was a lingering sense that "all things are possible" at any moment. But, growth usually takes time, flowers do not bud over night, and healing requires inner change within or without community. (Paul Solomon)

Collective interest, group prayer, and persistent efforts bring results when a true healing circle is created. But, when the time is right and preparation complete.

People used to ask the reader Edgar Cayce, "When will I be healed?" He would respond, "When you are ready for a new life? Will a healed body make you a better person? Will your healing make any difference to the people and the world around you?"

Bleeding Always Stops

Years ago when I was sitting with my father in his latter days at the same time I was passing through my own uncomfortable changes, I spoke to my friend JFK over the phone. Other friends had offered suggestions for remedies as well as their condolences on my dis- ease. But, Mr. K. gave me a favorite bit of wisdom as he said, "Bleeding always stops."

Those three words would be reassuring to very few. To me, they succinctly affirmed my own long held philosophies of trusting in the process, remembering Who holds the keys to life, and recalling that our single lives are but pearls on an endless string.

- There is rhyme and reason to every illness and injury, pain and trauma we suffer. Chaos only exists in the human imagination. Since we so often only see the surface of things, it can be difficult to understand "what is really going on." On down the road with the passage of time, we may get glimmers of light on the subject.
- Medicine and physicians have a place in modern society, but their services even when necessary and correct only act as instruments to inner forces and knowledge. The latter can make the best of bad practice and wrong decisions. In fact, "All things work for good" eventually and inevitably.
- Nature has more healing mechanisms than "Carter's got pills," as my mother might say. One of them is death.
- Death, like time and love, is a great healer. Many of us would like

to live on in fading bodies for centuries, but to what purpose, with what family, and what difference would it make to anyone but ourselves?

Death is just the ending of a cycle, a closure in the physical world, and re-entry "full-time" into inner worlds. Bleeding stops, the heart rests, and the body returns to ashes. The soul likewise goes back to its Source.

Death can cause gnashing of teeth and extended misery both to the dying one and to friends and family. Many people talk about going to heaven to be with God, but few are really prepared when the time comes. They hold on tightly. Fear produces pain. They may think they are ready for heaven, but eager volunteers are rare.

I remember my mother talking a few days before she died. Confined to bed for some time, she spoke about seeing a light coming into her room the night before. Mother hoped that it was a sign, but she also thought she might have fooled herself. Woefully, she said, "I wish I had religion." Religion may have helped, but it is no sure cure when we are facing the final passage. Or what we commonly call the final passage.

One of the greatest shortcomings of medicine - and religion – has been in regard to preparing people for death. The Christian church's response has been merely to tell people, "If you are saved, you will go to be with God." Medicine has avoided the issue entirely. Often medicating patients to such an extent that their passages may not be painful, but may be then at best totally unconscious blurs.

Conversely, various traditions give clear recommendations on how to prepare for the passage allowing the greatest amount of awareness at the time of death. Some day, these methods will be adopted in the West and help to clear the barrier between the worlds. In the meantime, there have been some encouraging movements on the edges of medicine if not in its very midst. Elisabeth Kubler-Ross did her original studies and wrote her thoughtful books on *Death and Dying* in the 70s. These helped to open many eyes, some of them belonging to medical professionals.

The Hospice Movement has been of great benefit to many, many families. To get support, help and respite as they care for members in the last weeks and months of life. Having experienced hospice with both my parents, I will opine that the concept is wonderful and the workers praiseworthy.

The administration of the program has come under medical control which seems to fit the era. But, death and dying are surely more natural than medical processes. Why do physicians have to be in charge? How many people have they held hands with when they were taking their last breaths?

My mother's passage to death was slow and inexorable after her breast cancer recurred and spread. She was in and out of the hospital and wanted to go again. Her surgeon, whom she respected, was kind enough to come to the house. He stood at the foot of her bed and told her, "There is nothing more we can do. You are better off here." Would that he had moved a few feet closer and held her hand when he said those words.

The whole family cared for mother until the last few days. Then hospice workers came in on regular visits. The family minister appeared from time to time. He came again on Good Friday, sat with her, and recited the 23rd Psalm. As he spoke, "Yea though I walk through the valley of the shadow of death, I will fear no evil," Mother breathed her final breath.

There is a prequel to this story. When Mother first developed breast cancer, the three sons living away from home were not told until after her mastectomy surgery. Her recovery went quickly although it took quite some time for her left arm to work as it used to. Three or four years later when I lived in Arizona, Mother recounted in her letters some of the events surrounding the recurrence of her cancer.

She had been prescribed a series of 33 radiation treatments to be done in a medical center 70 miles from home. Both parents were in their seventies when my father drove her on weekday trips for treatments. Midway through the ordeal, my father started having pains in his arms and eventually was taken to the local hospital with a heart attack.

He was apparently in serious condition for a few days. My mother went up to visit Dad after one of her treatments. She wrote in a letter to me: "I went to his bedside and asked him how he was doing. He didn't say much. Tight-lipped as usual. I told him, 'You can't kick the bucket now. You have to stay and take care of me.'" Dad recovered. Mother, who had been the caregiver for forty odd years, became the receiver. With help from the boys, Dad took up doing laundry, made some meals, put Mom in and out of bed and the bathtub. Some of the friction and frustrations of past years between the two melted away with roles reversed.

Mother's healing came with her death. Dad lived for 15 more years in which time he appeared as a different person. He became sociable. He was then a regular at the senior center, played pool with new cronies, and took off on summer bus tours. Over those years, his sons got the chance to know him on his own. Dad died when his time was up.

There will always be obstacles and pains and traumas in life. They do not happen haphazardly regardless of what we think. But, "It always works," as the bus-driving angel tells Robert Downey, Jr. in the waning moments of the spirited movie *Heart and Souls*.

It always works in the movies and it always works in real life. Even though things don't flow quite so quickly and smoothly in the mundane world as in Hollywood. Trust in God and Life.

IT ALWAYS WORKS.

Speaking of Hollywood, there is another film worthy of consideration with regard to the subject of life and death and dying. It is called *Whose Life Is It Anyway?* Starring Richard Dreyfuss, the film - first book, then play - tells the story of a quadriplegic on life support who sues to gain the right to end his own life. Against the standard ethic of "keep 'em alive at all costs," the story eventually confronts the key question.

There may be another layer to the issue worth considering. Whose Life Is It Anyway? deals with a man's own right to live or die. But, the title also belies another question as to whether we are really who we think we are. Aren't we really much more than we usually dare to imagine? Whose life are we living?

We are so used to bodily existence, using our thoughts, motivated by our feelings towards people and things and times. But, it is really the Soul's Life which we are living. We have that privilege and opportunity. Which also obliges us - if we are open and willing - to make the best of our time passing through this three-dimensional space. Doing so wisely makes the world a better place for everyone including ourselves on return visits.

An Inside Job

Most of the time medical practice is involved with getting rid of uncomfortable symptoms, disturbing cosmetic problems, and abnormal test results. When physicians are successful with their symptomatic therapy, they may pat themselves on the back. Their patients may be relieved, grateful, even happy.

But at best, only the surface of things has generally been affected. A "cure" may have been achieved, but at what cost and for how long? Will the problem recur or morph into another? Will the treatment come back to create more problems to deal with?

Application of treatment from outside the patient is usually just a beginning. Real involvement by the patient is almost always needed for real healing to occur, for a patient to rise to the next level and for the new self to begin to be born. Andrew Weil tells it the following way: "True healing can only take place through a change in consciousness, everything else is just therapy."

We need not dispense with therapy because it is "just therapy." It may in fact be the avenue through which a patient discovers needed information, has an "Aha" moment, is deeply moved by a therapist or practitioner, gets pointed in the right direction, is awakened or quickened toward needed change, is divested of a final outer impediment to fuller living.

Pain killers and chemical agents, surgery and radiation have their places. Although they will decrease in use as more physicians and patients turn toward substantive answers and deeper guidance. Standard practice will continue but include more subtle therapies in the likes of those used in anthroposophical medicine, homeopathy, Bach remedies, hands-on methods, energy work, etc.

Practitioners will not merely address their attention to the bodily shell by suppressing symptoms to "overwhelm the enemy." Since the conflict is really within, preparations will be prescribed which will attenuate symptoms allowing patients to watch them as they pass through. Consider their timing, value and meaning. And, come out the other side of an illness with some awareness and understanding of the process.

Steps in the direction of real healing will entail

- Engaging the family and community in the healing process. Illness happens in context of community. Resolution also needs to be found there as well.
- Practitioners and patients and families looking within. Beyond skin and bones, Xrays and blood to the emotional sphere, the mental body, and the soul. "Our soul exists in space and is inside us, like teeth in our mouth." (Boris Pasternak, *Dr. Zhivago*)
- Learning to make the best of standard medicine and join it with the same in alternative practices.
- Committing to study and research into the energetic nature of the human forms. Drawing on the knowledge of the ancients and the talents of modern seers and sensitives.
- Endeavoring to place illness in the context of time and life cycles. Practical astrology will help in coming days to show that human problems are relatively predictable. Furthermore, the astrological art will be valuable in giving a sense of how long ailments may last. "I can go through most anything, if I know how long it will take."
- Recognizing our station in time and space. Realizing that the body in which we live is one of many we have inhabited and will inhabit over eons of time. One third of physical existence is now spent away from the body during the hours of sleep. We pass much more time in the soul state between incarnations without any physical form.

- Realizing that embodiment is just for a moment, but recurs again and again. We only say "Goodbye" to our friends and enemies for periods. We will be back and so will they. So will our opportunities and problems return, dependent on how we live in this round.
- Addressing the fears of illness, pain and death. By pointing patients to their souls, inner relationships, and continuing existence, we begin to understand our place in the world, our responsibilities, and our possibilities.

ALL illness and injury results from some kind of inner friction, discontent and disharmony. If illness is an inside problem, so then healing is also an "inside job." Medicine is just beginning to spend time looking at real causes, studying the mind beyond the brain, imagining that man really has a soul. But, these efforts are sure to expand and bring valid and valuable results.

Moving in that direction, physicians will realize more fully what Dr. Albert Schweitzer recognized a century ago, "Each patient carries his own doctor inside." If the Doctor is already In, why do we persist searching for cures and healing on the outside?

All healing is really self healing. This simple concept is ancient and surely goes back long before Schweitzer and even Hippocrates, his bedside medicine, expectant manner, and credo that our natures are the real physicians. Belief in the healing power of nature, vis medicatrix naturae, must be recovered for the betterment of medicine and the multitude of patients who are its subjects.

I once consulted with a woman named Yolanda who had seen her husband killed before her eyes. Her husband was crushed to death between two vehicles. Yolanda was "crushed" as well. Soon after her husband's death, she developed an auto-immune disorder which manifested in pain and partial paralysis, inflammation and edema in her legs. Yolanda received orthodox medical therapy including cortisone and other anti-inflammatory drugs. Yet, she remained confined to a wheelchair and experienced recurring exacerbations of her disabling symptoms.

I asked her what she would do when she was healed. She replied, "I understand how it feels to be crippled. I will visit people in the hospital who are bedridden or stuck in a wheelchair. And I will go to church again."

I recommended that she begin to do those things right away, preparing for renewed health while she shared with others. I also suggested that if she could go to the hospital or clinic as a patient, she was able to go there as a visitor and a helper. Similarly, if she could find her way to medical appointments, she could make her way to church on Sunday. Acting AS IF can be an important part of the process of becoming well, being healed, achieving wholeness.

All healing is really self healing. The only question is about which self we invoke. How big is the Self? Still, it can be a big step to move from the old self to the new one, from the small to the greater Self.

Opportunities are waiting *patiently* in front of Yolanda and you and me. Whether we recognize them and put them to good use for ourselves and others becomes the big question. Physicians who came out of the Islamic tradition in the Middle Ages knew full well that, "God sends down no malady without also sending down with it a cure."

Yolanda, like all of us, had it inside her very being to pass through her trauma, grow out of adversity, and to vision a new self. That Self is, was and always will be found within.

The Greatest Healer

I had only the one meeting with Yolanda as she resided on the other side of the country and was visiting family in the Southwest when I saw her. That she found the resources and energy to travel across the USA suggested her potential to do more for herself and others.

I don't know if she ever took substantial steps towards conscious healing. I do remember one man who did. A quite amazing story was his, how he moved outside his routine, joined in community, and made extraordinary steps toward healing.

One summer in the 80s, a friend and I drove to the annual meeting of the Association for Holistic Health in San Diego. Because of Susan's previous involvement with the conference, we were able to sign up with fifty others for an intensive week-long workshop called the Health Optimizing Institute. I experienced HOI as a real high point in group sharing and interaction. A faculty of holistic authors and practitioners offered their stories, insights and visions with us throughout the week. They came to our meeting place rather than following the usual pattern of participants moving about the campus taking this class and that workshop. Several of the presenters rose above the rest and offered heart as well as mind as they demonstrated spirit at work in their lives.

But, the most effective teacher and learner of the week was a fellow participant who sat and listened quietly along with the rest of us. I only remember him speaking aloud in the group on two occasions. But, his words and sentiments and being came across powerfully.

I happened to stand in line next to Jack during the sign-in procedure on the first day of HOI. Outwardly, he was decidedly different from the rest of us. Jack was quadriplegic and had been so for 24 of his 42 years of life. He managed to get around on his own in a motorized wheelchair. But initially, Jack didn't get around to communicating in the group. His guard was up and he seemed quite distant and unapproachable. However, just his lone presence at this meeting seemed to make a quiet statement.

In the course of the week, whatever barriers he had carried with him vanished. Jack opened the door to his heart and people entered. He began to experience many of the interactions which he had missed in a life cloistered with his fawning mother over the past two and a half decades. Heart-to-heart became the flowing expression between Jack and the rest of us.

One day, Dr. Harold Bloomfield (psychiatrist and, at the time, author of a book on Transcendental Meditation) and his wife spent a couple hours with our group discussing and considering gems of wisdom from *A Course in Miracles*. At the end of their session which was held outside on the lawn of the SDSU campus, the Bloomfields led us in a meditation focused on The Miracle. When it was concluded,

Mrs. Bloomfield asked us to share what we thought a miracle was. There were a few silent moments before Jack's clear, deep voice penetrated the group with, "It's a miracle to be alive." There was no way to follow that response. We soon dispersed in a quiet, peaceful glow.

By the end of the week, Jack had become involved in many people's lives. He managed to participate in all group activities offered through HOI including the beach party held on the final evening of the program. Susan and I rode along in Jack's van as he drove to the beach north of San Diego. When we reached our destination, a foursome lifted Jack in his wheelchair over the sand dunes into the midst of the celebration. Jack was the center of attention for the whole of the occasion.

On the following day, the closing session occurred in which participants were each given an opportunity to express what HOI meant to them. Many stood up and shared how touched they were by the speakers, the program, and the group interactions. Tears flowed freely during those final moments, but most especially when Jack had his turn.

He told us, "I came here with a chip on my shoulder. I had been angry and frustrated for many years because of my lot in life. But somehow without my ever suspecting it, my heart melted and the chip fell off. As the week wore on, I knew I was being healed. I now know that I can go home and change my relationship with my poor old mom. Instead of fighting with her, I can love her now.

"Today, I feel a lot like the crippled man in the Bible story - the one who was lowered with his pallet through the roof into the presence of Jesus. The Master told the man his sins were forgiven and to take up his pallet and walk. That man was healed and walked home. Well, I got part of the deal. I can't get up and walk home today. But, it really doesn't matter. You know, how my body works just doesn't matter ... because I've been healed on the inside."

What a spine-tingling statement that was. What final lessons might we take from Jack's experience?

- Community can make a real difference in the healing process.

- Healing can happen any time, any place.

- Healing can take place in one moment or may take a lifetime. Or even longer.

- If we want to speed up our healing process, we may have to move out of our routine into the flow of a healing environment or help create it right where we live.

- Healing of body is only one aspect of the process, and often of lesser importance than our inner parts.

- Healing is really a communal venture. Energies are constantly circulating within a person, out and around and back. When they are purified and properly directed healing results.

- Healing self and healing others are the same. We are all connected.

All of the great traditions of the world have the Golden Rule in common, although stated in a variety of ways. "Do unto others" is merely an alternative version of "Love one another."

Which inevitably leads us to the Great Commandment of western tradition: "Love the Lord thy God with all thy heart, soul and mind, and thy neighbor as thyself."

Here is something about which we all can become enthusiastic. Love is surely the Great Healer. "God is Love." We are created in the image and likeness of that One. Being, living, expressing Love is the surest means to health and healing and reforming medicine. In whatever measure we can mobilize it, let us be about that work.

Afterword

Medicine and the media put the spotlight on disease, the urgency to tend to ill health, and the never ending struggle for cures. But it may have become clearer to the reader by now that in a substantial majority of times, our dis-ease is a conflict of internal energies which will inevitably move to resolution. We can get in the way or support the healing process. Dis-ease and healing are two sides of the same coin.

If we take the simplistic approach that all discomfort is unworthy of us and must be vanquished, we will certainly continue to keep physicians busy, spend much time in chasing cures, and delay our own growth into newer beings. But, we assuredly have the potential to grow and expand upward and inward to the unending source of Light, Love, and Life.

Let's close with a few final suggestions from Frugal Physician to Prudent Patients in the time of need:

- **Use Common Sense**. Medicine and physicians are at their best in delivering First Aid in time of emergency. Utilize them sparingly. True emergencies are rare.
- **Be Patient**. Nature (God) created you and your body in the course of nine months. Illness and injury eventuate over time - though it may seem otherwise - from the inside out. Realize that dis-ease and healing processes may take comparable periods of time to move from the inside out.
- **Be Smart**. Use your dis-ease and pain as learning opportunities. We are always meeting self and illness is one of the best ways to bring us to better understanding of who we are, why we came here, and what our purpose is.
- **Be Enthusiastic**. Put your mind and heart on important things. Dwelling on problems energizes them. Instead, let's seek re-sol-ution by focusing on the soul (sol) of things, give and grow, live and love as much as possible. Dis-ease may not go away quickly, but wholeness and health will surely grow in the background.

*The seed of God is in us.
Nut seeds grow into nut trees,
Pear seeds into pear trees,
And God seed into God.*

Meister Eckhardt

APPENDICES

Superficial & Subtle Body Energies

Acupuncture Meridians

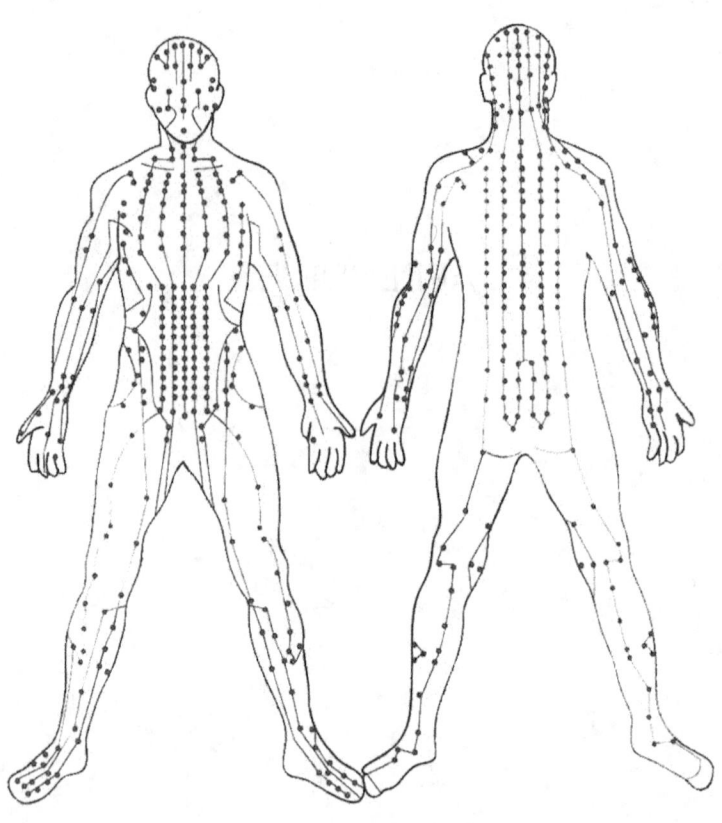

Mental-Emotional Energy Streams

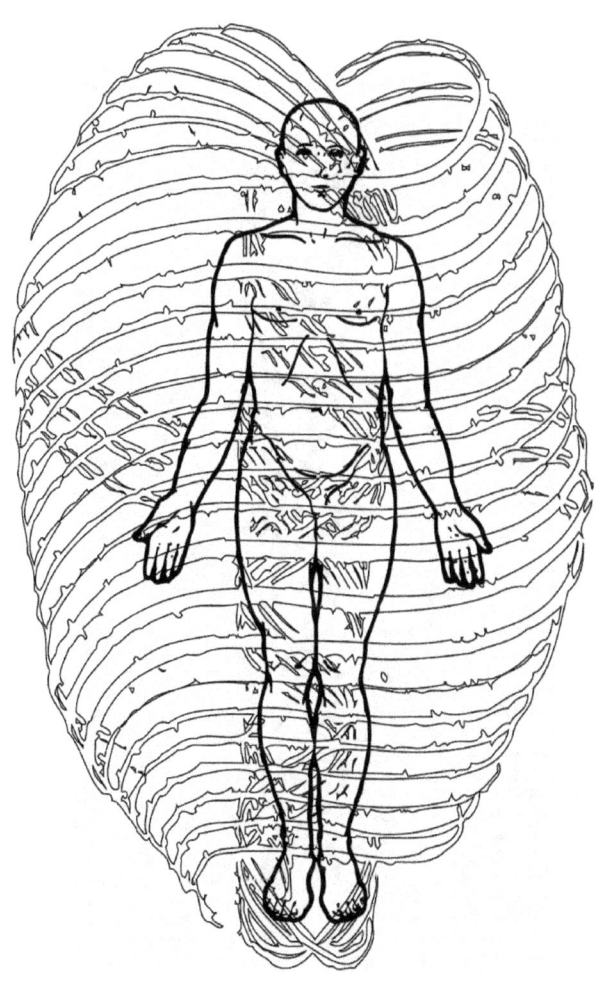

Psycho-Neuro-Endocrine System

Chakras

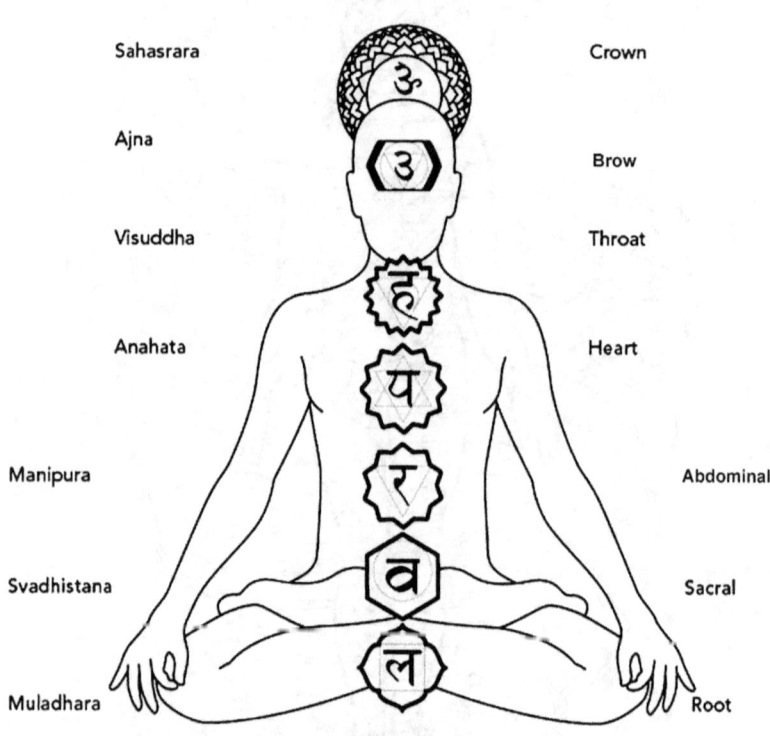

The seven major chakras in the body.

Endocrine – Centers

Nervous

Brain & Nerve Centers		Endocrine Glands
Cortex		Pineal
Midbrain		Pituitary
Cervical		Thyroid
Cardiac		Thymus
Solar		Pancreas
Pelvic		Gonads
Sacral		Adrenals

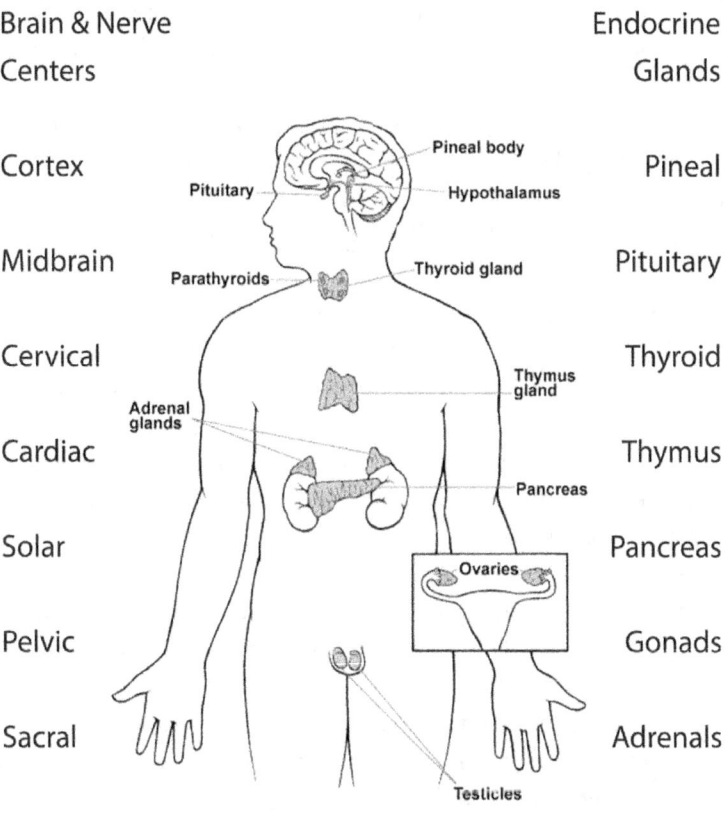

Hippocratic Oath - Original

I swear by Apollo, the healer, Asclepius, Hygeia, and Panacea, and I take to witness all the gods, all the goddesses, to keep according to my ability and my judgment, the following Oath and agreement:

To consider dear to me, as my parents, him who taught me this art; to live in common with him and, if necessary, to share my goods with him; To look upon his children as my own brothers, to teach them this art.

I will prescribe regimens for the good of my patients according to my ability and my judgment and never do harm to anyone.

I will not give a lethal drug to anyone if I am asked, nor will I advise such a plan; and similarly I will not give a woman a pessary to cause an abortion.

But I will preserve the purity of my life and my arts.

I will not cut for stone, even for patients in whom the disease is manifest; I will leave this operation to be performed by practitioners, specialists in this art.

In every house where I come I will enter only for the good of my patients, keeping myself far from all intentional ill-doing and all seduction and especially from the pleasures of love with women or with men, be they free or slaves.

All that may come to my knowledge in the exercise of my profession or in daily commerce with men, which ought not to be spread abroad, I will keep secret and will never reveal.

If I keep this oath faithfully, may I enjoy my life and practice my art, respected by all men and in all times; but if I swerve from it or violate it, may the reverse be my lot.

Oath of Maimonides

The eternal providence has appointed me to watch over the life and health of Thy creatures. May the love for my art actuate me at all time; may neither avarice nor miserliness, nor thirst for glory or for a great reputation engage my mind; for the enemies of truth and philanthropy could easily deceive me and make me forgetful of my lofty aim of doing good to Thy children.

May I never see in the patient anything but a fellow creature in pain.

Grant me the strength, time and opportunity always to correct what I have acquired, always to extend its domain; for knowledge is immense and the spirit of man can extend indefinitely to enrich itself daily with new requirements.

Today he can discover his errors of yesterday and tomorrow he can obtain a new light on what he thinks himself sure of today.

Oh, God, Thou has appointed me to watch over the life and death of Thy creatures; here am I ready for my vocation and now I turn unto my calling.

The Doctor and The Prince

By George Bernard Shaw

Once upon a time, in the country of the Half Mad, which was cut off from the western end of Europe in prehistoric times to prevent the inhabitants from injuring any but themselves, the King fell ill. As he had always been well spoke of, and had established very kindly relations with his subjects, his illness caused a great increase of their affection for him and his family. All the married women saw in the Queen a wife anxious about her husband, with a sick-bed to provide for. All the men saw in the King a fellow-man suffering as they themselves had suffered or might at any moment have to suffer. For sickness is a Great Leveller, and consequently a great breeder of sympathy added to loyalty, the nation was in such a state of concern about the King as had never before arisen within living memory. Naturally, the case being one of dangerous illness, it was to the doctors that the nation turned for help and reassurance.

Now in the country of the Half Mad the doctors had long before this taken the place of the medieval Church. There was a law that when a man was ill he must on pain of punishment send for his parish priest; but this law had been so long disregarded that only a few specialists in Church history knew of its existence. Its place had been taken by a law that when there was sickness in the house the doctor must be sent for, and that if the doctor said that any part of a sick child's body must be cut out its parent must have that done at once whether they approved or not, or else be haled before a magistrate and heavily fined, or, should the child have died, committed for having killed it.

To such powers as this were added extraordinary privileges. For instance, doctors were licensed to commit murder with impunity, provided they did it either administering poison or by using knives of a particular shape in such a manner that the victim did not die until he or she had been put in bed. Not only was no inquest held and no indictment brought against the do, but he was actually paid for his labor, and sometimes invited to the funeral.

As the Half Mad were so jealous of their liberties that a priest could not even order a father to have his child baptized, it will be seen that this strange people, though half sane on the subject of priests, were wholly mad on the subject of doctors, willingly granting them powers which they had denied to their Kings at the cost of revolution and civil war.

Now the doctors, being no worse than other people, did their best to prove worthy of their extraordinary trust by using it for the relief of the sick, and making it impossible for anyone to become a doctor except by years of study to qualify him for his duties. But as the Half Mad, whilst bowing down with the deepest reverence to the condition of conscience which they supposed these studies to confer, would not pay a doctor anything until they were actually ill and threatened with death, the doctors were mostly poor, and would have starved altogether if the nation had been in a reasonably healthy condition. Thus their duty to themselves and their wives and children was to keep their patients ill as long and as often as possible; to persuade them that they were dangerously ill when there was nothing the matter with them that their recuperative powers could not cure; and even to deprive them of as many of their limbs and organs as they could without killing the goose that laid the golden eggs. On the other hand, their duty to their parents and their country was to do exactly the contrary, and strive to their utmost to produce a state of things in which doctors would starve.

Now in the kingdom of the Half Mad, people always ended by believing what they wanted to believe, no matter how much it might be contradicted by facts; and so it had come about that the doctors, though they were as kindly and honorable as could reasonably be expected, and sometimes very clever, had built up an elaborately reasoned ingenious series of mechanical explanations of all the diseases, giving them impressive names, and setting forth the treatments and operations and medicines proper to them, until at last they could do almost anything with a patient except cure him or even allow him a fair chance of curing himself. Thus the calling of a doctor to the sick-bed was rather a pious ceremony enforced by law that a proceeding from which any relief to the patient could be expected. But the patient would die in their hands; and this was very necessary for the settlement of the affairs of the patient who had any affairs to settled.

With a Faith (for such it was) in this condition, naturally there were Heresies in all directions. New methods of treating disease were discovered; but the doctors took so long to learn the old ones that they had not time for new ones. Even the surgeons had to do without any manual training and picked up their art as the father of a family picks up the art of carving a turkey. So, instead of adopting the new methods, they excommunicated the new practitioners and all their accomplices. Only, as the heretics either cured their patients or at least did not kill them by obsolete and barbarous treatments, the doctors, when they were ill themselves, often resorted to the heretics for treatment.

This was the state of things when the King fell ill. He had twelve doctors to attend him; and when there was no sign of his being cured, his people became anxious and said, "A single doctor is generally sufficient to kill one of us, so how can the King survive twelve doctors?"

Then the King's son, who was at the other side of the world among the black savages (for he was very tired of the white ones), came flying, sailing, and express-training at an amazing speed back to his father, and spoke with the King's chief physician, who was so delightful a person that his patients were often cured by his mere appearance in the bedroom. The Prince knew that the father's case must be most serious since it resisted the presence of this great healer and the influence of the King's faith in him.

And the Prince said to him: "Doc, the King my father does not seem to be getting any better. Is it not possible to get a move on?"

"In what direction, sir?" replied the chief physician.

"In the direction of getting him up and about," said the Prince.

"Everything is being done that can properly be done," said the physician. "If your Royal Highness has not confidence in our knowledge and devotion --"

"Stow that," said the Prince. "Your devotion is all right, but your knowledge is bunk."

"Bunk!" exclaimed the chief physician, highly scandalized.

"Well, perhaps not all of it," said the Prince, feeling that he had gone a little too far, "but I cannot help knowing what everyone knows, and that is that according to your own best men nine-tenths of your official notions are fit only for the dustbin. I have a heap of letters, books, pamphlets, and magazines here which have been sent me; and they have disturbed me very much."

"I have not read these documents," said the physician. "If your Royal Highness can suggest any measure we have omitted, my opinion is at your service."

"Drugs, now?" said the Prince. "Drugs are bunk, are they not?"

"Undoubtedly, from a purely secular point of view, drugs are bunk," said the physician, "but in the case of a royal patient I could not possibly take the responsibility of withholding form His Majesty the official remedies from our materia medica."

"But," said the Prince, "there is a way of giving drugs in infinitesimal quantities to which all the latest discoveries and scientific speculations point as the right way."

"Infinitesimals," replied the physician, "are used only by homeopaths: that is, by empirics who, being ignorant of the nature of disease, merely treat its symptoms. If you bring a Chinese patient to a homeopath, he will treat him for yellow fever."

"Do you really know the nature of disease any more than a homeopath does?" said the Prince.

"Certainly," said the physician. "I have passed an examination in pathology, and written books about it. What a strange question!"

"What is the nature of my father's complaint?" said the Prince.

"It is what we call pleurisy," said the physician.

"I know that," said the Prince. "I know its name; and I know it symptoms. What is its nature?"

"If I knew that," said the physician, "perhaps I could cure it."

"Then pathology is bunk," said the Prince, who had picked up this expression from a famous motor-car manufacturer, who had applied to History. "Let us call in a homeopath."

"Unfortunately," said the physician, "the only one in London whose reputation and success would satisfy public opinion has not been admitted to our communion; and if I discussed the case with him I should be excommunicated."

"Well," said the Prince, "they say a lot of trouble comes from spinal displacements. What about my father's spine?"

"It looks all right," said the physician.

"But there are chaps who are trained to feel whether it is all right or not," said the Prince. "There is a machine that will register on a galvanometer displacement that nobody can feel."

"I never heard of it," said the physician. "I can assure you that these people who feel spines are almost all ignorant Americans who have spent two years in mere manual training instead of in the study of pathology."

"All the same," said the Prince, "they bring off cures occasionally; so why not call one in?"

"I should be excommunicated if I were seen speaking to one," said the physician.

"Why not do it yourself?" said the Prince. "You are a surgeon."

"I have not had the two years' training," said the physician, "it is not part of our official surgery."

"Official surgery is a wash-out," said the Prince. "What about testing my father's blood for radiation? That can be done by a rheostat, can't it? And there is some method of neutralizing the rays that sometimes cures, isn't there?"

"But it was discovered by an American," said the physician.

"I am prepared to overlook that if my father's health can be restored by this method," said the Prince.

"Impossible," said the physician. "He was not only an American, but a Jew."

"I understand he was a proper doctor all the same," persisted the Prince.

"No doubt," said the physician, "but the treatment would involve attaching His Majesty to the electric light switch; and public opinion would never tolerate that."

"Public opinion be blowed!" said the Prince. "Do you suppose I am going to let my father lose a chance because people are fools? Besides, we can use a private battery."

"It may not be," said the physician. "This discovery reached us only about a dozen years ago, and is not yet recognized by our Vatican. I dare not take the responsibility of experimenting on the King with a treatment that has not been proved by at least fifty years' experience."

"Proved to do what?" said the Prince. "To cure the disease?"

"To have stood the test of being taught in our medical schools as the logical and appropriate treatment," said the physician.

"Do the patients recover under your logical and appropriate treatment?" said the Prince.

"Sometimes," said the physician. "Quite frequently."

"They might do that if they had no treatment at all," said the Prince.

"That is true," said the physician. "The recuperative power of the human organism is marvellous. Quacks take advantage of that, I am sorry to say."

"I am not satisfied about all this," said the Prince. "It seems to me that my father, just because he is a king, is cut off from the benefit of all the new discovers and treatments that are available for the meanest of his subjects."

"I exhort your Royal Highness to be patient," said the physician. "Your royal father is in the hands of God."

"You mean that we should call in a Christian Science practitioner?" said the Prince.

"Most certainly not," said the physician. "I and my colleagues would be obliged to withdraw at once if such a person were admitted to the palace."

"Another wash-out," said the Prince.

"Not at all, said the physician. "We should not object to a visit from His Majesty's domestic chaplain; though of course we could not allow him to treat the case; and anything in the nature of a consultation would be out of the question."

"In short," said the Prince, "my poor father is in the hands of your confounded Vatican. However, I suppose we must make the best of it. I should like to call in your Pope for a consultation."

"We should have to tell him what to say beforehand," said the physician. "You see, he was qualified more than half a century ago, and may not be quite up to date."

"But I have looked him up in Who's Who," said the Prince, "and he has ninety distinctions and qualifications, entitling him to a dozen medical letters after his name. I attach great importance to a lot of letters because I have nothing else to go by."

"As I myself have only six, you naturally consider his opinion twice as valuable as mine," said the physician.

"Well, if the letters don't mean that, they don't mean anything," said the Prince.

"Precisely," said the physician.

"Then your Pope is another wash-out," said the Prince. "Are there any laymen on your Vatican council to represent my father and all the other patients?"

"A notorious enemy of our profession has succeeded, after years of agitation, in having one layman appointed," said the Prince.

"Officially, no," said the physician.

"But unofficially -- as between man and man?" pleaded the Prince.

"Since your Royal Highness is good enough to admit me to that footing," said the physician, "I am bound to say, as between man and man, that the exclusion of laymen from a body whose business it is to safeguard the general interests of the laity against the sectional interests of the medical profession is only one out of the many instances of the almost incredible incapacity of the Half Mad for taking care of themselves. In respect of the art of life, our people must be set aside as unqualified practitioners."

"This is a world of bunk," said the Prince, "and the boasted capacity of my father's subjects for self-government is the biggest bunk of the lot. But my father's life is in danger. I appeal to you to throw over your silly Vatican and be a friend to us in our need. If they give you the sack you shall have a dukedom and a pension of a hundred thousand a year. Tell me what is the most up-to-date scientific treatment for my father?"

"I have already ordered it," said the physician. "And you will be glad to hear it will involve no conflict on my part with my colleagues."

"Splendid!" said the Prince. "I will never forget this proof of your sympathy and devotion. What is the treatment?"

"The seaside," said the physician.

"The seaside!" cried the Prince. "You call that the latest! Why, it is what my great-grandmother would have recommended."

"Yes," said the physician, "but not for the true scientific reason. She thought that benefit arose from change of air."

"Then what does it arise from? said the Prince.

"That," said the physician, "is a professional secret which I can impart to you only under a solemn pledge that it shall go no further."

"I give you my word of honor," said the Prince. "What will the seaside really do to cure my father?"

The physician stooped to the Prince's ear, and whispered. "It will get him away from the doctors."

Shortly afterwards, the king recovered.

Bibliography & References

Adams, Patch. *Gesundheit*. Healing Arts Press: Rochester, VT, 1998.
Andrews, Michael. *The Life That Lives on Man*. Arrow: London, UK, 1976.
Avalon, Arthur. *The Serpent Power*. Dover Publications: NY, NY, 1974.
Bach, Edward. *Heal Thyself*. C.W. Daniel Co: Essex, England, 1987.
Bailey, Alice. *Esoteric Healing*. Lucis Publishing Company: NY, NY, 1953.
Barasch, Marc Ian. *The Healing Path*. Arkana Penguin: NY, NY, 1993.
Becker, Robert. *The Body Electric*. Morrow: New York 1985.
Becker, Rollin. "Diagnostic Touch: Its Principles and Application." *AAO Yearbook*, 1963.
Carrel, Alexis. *Man, The Unknown*. Harper and Brothers: NY, NY, 1935.
Cayce, Edgar. *Readings*. Edgar Cayce Foundation: Virginia Beach, VA, 1977.
Cousins, Norman. *Anatomy of an Illness*. Norton and Co: NY, NY, 1979.
Dixon, Bernard. *Powers Unseen*. W.H. Freeman & Co: NY, NY, 1994.
Dossey, Larry. *Space, Time and Medicine*. Shambhala: Boulder, CO, 1984.
Frankl, Viktor. *Man's Search for Meaning*. Washington Square Press: NY, NY, 1965.
Govinda, Lama. *Foundations of Tibetan Mysticism*. Weiser: NY, NY, 1975.
Grossinger, Richard. *Planet Medicine*. Doubleday Anchor: NY, NY, 1989.
Howard, Philip K. *The Death of Common Sense*. Grand Central Publishing: NY, NY, 1995.
Jung, Carl (editor). *Man and His Symbols*. Dell Publishing: NY, NY, 1982.
Illich, Ivan. *Medical Nemesis*. Random House: NY, NY, 1976.
Mead, G.R.S. *The Doctrine of the Subtle Body*. Theosophical Publishing House: Wheaton, IL, 1967.
Mendelsohn, Robert. *Confessions of a Medical Heretic*. Warner Books: NY, NY, 1979.
Millard, Margaret. *Casebook of a Medical Astrologer*. Weiser: NY, NY, 1980.
Oyle, Irving. *The Healing Mind*. Celestial Arts: Milbrae, CA, 1974.
Penfield, Wilder. *The Mystery of the Mind*. Princeton University Press: Princeton, NJ, 1975.
Peck, M. Scott. *A Different Drum*. Simon and Schuster: NY, NY, 1987.
Pert, Candace. *"Neuropeptides: Emotions and Bodymind."* Noetic Sciences Review, Sausalito, CA, 1987.
Porter, Roy. *The Greatest Benefit to Mankind*. WW Norton: NY, NY, 1997.

Sheldrake, Rupert. *A New Science of Life*. Tarcher: Los Angeles, CA, 1981.
Selzer, Richard. *Mortal Lessons*. Simon and Schuster: NY, NY, 1976.
Siegel, Bernie. *Love, Medicine and Miracles*. Harper & Row: NY, NY, 1977.
Thomas, Lewis. *The Medusa and the Snail*. Penguin: NY, NY, 1995.
Watson, Lyall. *Lifetide*. Hodder and Stoughton: London, England, 1979.
Weil, Andrew. *Health and Healing*. Houghton Mifflin: Boston, MA, 1983.

The Doctor and The Prince is by George Bernard Shaw, 1929

All Images: Public Domain or Creative Commons CC0 1.0 Universal. Please contact The Portable School Press with any attribution issues. Thank you image creators.

About The Author

Robert McNary is an erstwhile physician who learned more about health and healing after he left medicine than during his twenty years in training and working in the field. Healing is as big as life itself. Medicine is a small but vital part of the larger world of healing. However, most healing, like life, occurs away from the hospital and doctors' offices. We ALL need to become more conscious and active in the work of healing.

Dr. Bob has not practiced medicine for decades but considers himself more a doctor now than when he wore a white coat. Doctor originally meant Teacher, and teaching doctors are sorely needed so that the People can recover Medicine and Healing. Dr. Bob believes a new/old paradigm of healing must arise in the near time to complement and supplement physician-oriented, technological, business-based medicine. That broad form of healing will combine community consciousness and the gift of healing hands. Everyone's!

Robert has written a number of books, most notably *Baby Doctor* and *PHENOMENON: 13 Lives of the Millennium Man*. He is presently working on a series of books on a universal healing method practiced in the 18th and 19th centuries. It has important lessons for the present day. When not writing or researching, Bob spends his life walking the country and discovering extraordinary people and places.

PEOPLE MEDICINE

is more than a book.

It is an opportunity for continued learning and networking through associated website: **peoplemedicine.net,** a monthly electronic newsletter and email contact with author.

Visit our website to

• Learn about Prudent Patients and Frugal Physicians,
• Share your own story, perspectives and brainstorms,
• Keep up with the latest news about People Medicine.
• Sign up for our newsletter

After you have read the book,
feel free to send comments to the author at
theportableschool@gmail.com

~~~~~~~~

Contact us about our other books/products:

Baby Doctor
Montana Made Me Do It
Phenomenon
Pictorial Astrology

Visit our other websites:
rockymountainastrologer.com
theportableschool.com
phenom1000man.com

The Portable School Press
theportableschool@gmail.com

www.ingramcontent.com/pod-product-compliance
Lightning Source LLC
Chambersburg PA
CBHW050616300426
44112CB00012B/1528